HOW NOT
TO TEACH YOGA

Lessons on Boundaries,
Accountability, and Vulnerability

– Learnt the Hard Way

TORI LUNDEN

Dedicated to any teacher who has ever stood at the front of a yoga class and thought, "What the hell am I doing?"

Contents

Acknowledgements

I am indebted to the ancient tradition of Yoga along with the Indian masters and practitioners who, despite colonial persecution, kept this diverse tradition alive so that people like myself can benefit from its wisdom today. It is my hope that the practices presented in this book help create more opportune conditions for the wisdom of this tradition to be shared and learned.

I recognize and thank all my teachers—past and present, formal and informal—in yoga, social work, and life. Your influence has propelled me forward and, to paraphrase a favourite prayer of mine from Christianity, "Thank-you for bringing me to where I did not want to be." Special thanks to my Advaita Vedanta teacher and to my therapist—while seemingly at odds, together you are a winning combination.

Finally, heartfelt thanks to my parents, Anita and Neil, who while I was growing up always prompted me to, "Maybe think about that a little more," whenever I came home with an easy, dogmatic answer about life, spirituality, or other people. And who afforded me nothing but respect and freedom when I told them in 2008 I was giving up a promising career in social work to go study Yoga in India.

Introduction:
Teaching Yoga Is Hard

I didn't want to teach the class.

I was doing it as a solid for another teacher. Her class at the studio was immediately after mine and she was stuck in traffic, afraid she wouldn't make it in time. I didn't especially want to teach again that Sunday afternoon, particularly not for her. She inspired a sort of righteous devotion in her students that I found distasteful...while simultaneously being jealous of her class numbers. But we were friends, in a fake church lady way, so I texted back, "Of course, babe."

Her students were fairly good about it. Meaning none of them turned and walked out the door after hearing the news. We were about to start when she burst into the studio with a triumphant, "I'm here! I made it!" The whole class cheered. A woman I had just signed in exclaimed, "Oh thank God!" as she turned and made direct eye contact with me.

There was an awkward pause.

"Thank you so much for offering to teach, Tori! Everyone, isn't Tori fab?"

She glided past me into the studio and off they all went to samadhi, leaving me conspicuously behind to find my own, fab way out the front door

Outside in the parking lot, I debated keying her car.

Seriously, Teaching Yoga Is Hard

Let's just take a moment to really acknowledge this before we move on to anything else.

Teaching yoga is hard and we all occasionally doubt our ability to do it well. And how could we not?

For starters, we have all of the different styles and theories of how to approach this colossal thing called Yoga; we have all of the different, and sometimes conflicting, new research on how best to work with our bodies/minds/emotions/breath; we have our own personal experiences that we bring with us to the front of the classroom; we have the social context of living in a post-colonial world; don't forget commodification and the yoga industrial complex; and then, THEN, we have putting all of that together into some kind of cohesive offering for a classroom full of unique individuals.

Put it that way and damn right we all have imposter syndrome. Who is capable of doing all that in 75 minutes?

On top of all that we have to figure how exactly we choose to execute this feat of multitasking. In sorting out the nuts and bolts of sequencing, cueing, demoing, etc., we often, and easily, overlook in what spirit we are conveying this information. We are told to be authentic and to find our own voice but we are given very few (if any) tools to help us do this in an effective and safe way. Most 200 hour teacher trainings are already bursting with so much information, that the" how" of teaching often gets left out. Yoga Philosophy, while amazing as framework for living, does little to help us figure out the practicalities of how to offer that same amazing information to others.

It's a common trap among yoga teachers: we learn how to engage with bodies, but not necessarily how to skillfully engage with people. As a result, we often fall into either interacting with our students the same way we would with friends and family members, and/or we copy the mannerisms and techniques of our own teachers. It's a bit like parenting in that way. Neither of these is inherently a bad thing, but it can be a little like the blind leading the blind. If we have little to no personal boundaries with our family, chances are we won't have professional boundaries with our students. If our favourite teacher pretended to know everything there was to know about yoga while bypassing all ugly human emotions, then we will likely try do the same when we become a teacher. At one end of the spectrum we get too friendly and can't maintain healthy boundaries with students and at the other we get pseudo-gurus who teach from a place of contrived authority.

In my case, figuring out the dos and don'ts of teaching has been done largely through messing up time and time again. I graduated with a degree in Social Work long before I started teaching but that education and experience was something I put on the shelf when I decided to commit to yoga as a vocation. Partly because I was looking for a fresh start, and partly because it took repeatedly messing up to be able to appreciate how the best practices commonly found in social work could benefit both myself as a teacher and those in my classes. "Best Practices" simply means the best things we can do professionally to show up for ourselves and others. They are ideal behaviours and attitudes that we shoot for, knowing full well that we will most likely mess them up from time to time. What I present here is a model for teaching based on best practices as they apply to teaching yoga, in person or online. This isn't a book about what you teach, that's entirely up to you, it's about how you go about the art of teaching. Vinyasa Flow or Dru, best practices can be applied.

I share a lot of my own screw-up stories along the way because I really want to illustrate that these "how not tos" are not just things other teachers do. It'd be easy to write a book about everything I think is wrong with yoga but there wouldn't be much point in doing so other than bolstering a sense of moral superiority within me and those who happen to agree with me. It's easy to sit around and gossip about what everyone else gets wrong but the real work of honing our teaching skills comes from taking that gaze inward. We all screw up and we all usually do it while trying our darnedest to get it right.

This book is not about getting a correct answer to add to the pile of correct answers we already have. More information isn't helpful if we haven't done the work of learning how to apply it. If it was, none of us would have imposter syndrome, would we? Getting into how and why unhealthy teaching practices occur, or could potentially occur, means getting into the messiness that is in the roots of why we wanted to teach in the first place and why we want to be perfect at it now. It might suck a bit at times, but it's worth it. To help you with that, throughout the book there are exercises and questions to get you thinking about your own experiences and the ways you can incorporate these new concepts and practices into your own teaching style. The point of all this is never to make you teach like me, it's to give you tools to teach more reliably as yourself.

As we go through this, the point is never to make you feel bad. It's also not about making me feel bad—I'm self-critical in this book not out of shame but out of having enough self-love to own my past. Screwing up is part of the learning process and teaching is a learning process. Accountability to ourselves and our students is one of the most loving things we can do. We just need to remember to do it with compassion.

Okay. Here we go, but first say it with me one more time: "teaching yoga is hard."

A Few Things First

This practice sections of the book are purposely lacking in yoga philosophy. This is not because this topic is not relevant or worthy of study; it's because philosophy is not my area of expertise. I've been studying it for over a decade now but still consider myself a novice so I'm not going to give many lessons in that regard. Maybe I'll write a workbook for philosophy through the lens of interpersonal and social dynamics someday, but I'm not there yet so I'm sticking to what I know (more on that in the section on scope of practice).

As you read this, I ask that you keep in mind that my personal story is never the lesson; my stories are here only to help illustrate the lesson in an interesting way and are never a prescription for what your experience should be. What I present here is not the unbiased truth, because 1) that would be dry and analytical, and 2) unbiased truth doesn't exist outside of enlightenment and I'm not enlightened (spoiler). That my opinion creeps in is not a bad thing, but it needs to be acknowledged. The country I live in, my skin colour, my gender identity, socio-economic status, the types of yoga I have studied/taught and many other factors all influence the experiences I have had as a teacher, as do yours. This is another reason for an emphasis on you telling your story throughout the book. Your story is not only just as relevant as mine, it is bound to be different with its own unique challenges and insights.

One more thing on that—there are layers upon layers of nuance to everything covered in this book and I can't touch on all of it. If I have not addressed something that is important to you or a path of inquiry you want to go down, please do so on your own. Again, and I can't stress this enough, *I want you to make this work for you*, not me or some idealized version of teaching based on these practices. Social work theory and practices, like any human construct, are not without their flaws. The profession itself has a long and sordid history of causing harm under the guise of helping. And while the profession has sought to own and learn from these mistakes, it is undeniable that social work's history continues to influence how it is practiced today.

Self-Doubt:
We All Got It

Let's start with something we can all relate to: self-doubt. I'll come out and say it right now: what we discuss here might make you briefly feel worse about being a teacher before it helps you feel better. The cost of increased awareness is that things always seem to get worse simply because we are finally noticing what's really going on. Ignorance can be bliss temporarily, but then it usually comes back to bite us and those around us.

Self-doubt has been there my whole life. It's here right now as I'm writing this and will still be there when you read it. It's the voice in the back of my head telling me that whatever I think/do/teach/am is somehow wrong or not good enough. I likely don't have to tell you, it's a bit of bitch to deal with. When I started teaching, my self-doubt seemed to grow exponentially overnight. Not because there was more of it, but because I thought doing yoga meant self-doubt was supposed to disappear. It's all love and light until you show up to sub a class and everyone looks so pained at your not being their regular teacher that it's all you can do not to hide in the props cupboard to avoid their disappointed, judgmental gaze. Let's not kid ourselves, to feel doubt is to be human.

I have never met a single yoga teacher who didn't doubt themselves. I doubt such a teacher even exists...if they do, they are the last person on earth I would want to learn from. I don't trust people who don't question themselves occasionally. As such, I've stopped seeing doubt as the enemy we often make it out to be.

But, why do so many of us feel so insecure about teaching yoga? Well, in my opinion, these are the five major reasons:

1) Chances are that anyone who stands in front of a group for any reason has some pre-existing insecurities. Nothing wrong with that! It's called being human. Megalomaniac teachers like Bikram make the news but I think there are far more teachers out there who are simply introverts or highly sensitive people trying to connect with others via teaching. The implicit boundaries of the teacher/student dynamic can ease social anxieties for someone who normally struggles in groups, but it's not necessarily a sustainable solution.

2) Yoga can and does change lives. That's huge. That's also intimidating. After my first teacher training and subsequent teaching failure (more on that soon), I didn't teach or practice for six months because I couldn't handle the pressure of each and every movement and position being a means of healing and ecstatic bliss. What if I got it wrong and it backfired? Would my prana misfire and I'd never poop again?! I'm exaggerating a little but not much. Whatever focus your teaching and practice has, it can be overwhelming. Yoga is often seen as a universal cure-all but who among us is truly capable of curing anyone and everything? No one, but that's what we are sold. Which bring us to number 3.

3) Yoga became popular. There were more yoga teachers and more yoga studios...which created training programs and created more teachers...who opened more studios and created training programs. The market became saturated and it became competitive. We all started marketing ourselves and the best way to market seemed to be

creating the perfect yoga image (also a nice way of masking self doubt points #1 and #2). Then, specializations started emerging. More and more trainings and education were marketed. Most of them look really interesting and beneficial. All of them tell us how their information will make us a better teacher (subtext, we're less of a teacher without it). And maybe they're right, and most likely we all do need to be constantly learning, but good lord that's a lot of pressure coming from every which way on social media. It's so easy for that messaging to slip under the skin and be taken personally.

4) We also live in this thing called a society, and this society has norms that tell us some traits are desirable and others are not; all based on the insidious belief that there is only one correct way to be human. Only one way to get this whole life thing right. How limiting and anxiety-provoking is that to live with when it gets internalized? Let alone the increased limitations society tries to put on you the further away you are from this made-up ideal. That ideal being light skinned, heterosexual, cis-gendered, with the appearance of what is considered physically and mentally healthy. This is commonly known as privilege. If you're newer to this concept there's links to people who can teach you more in the "People to Follow and Learn From" section at the back of the book. For the purpose of this section, I'll leave it at this: while the categorization of traits as desirable and undesirable is not inherently true, the consequences of living in a society that believes in this hierarchy is very much real.

5) This one is yours. What do you see as a major reason for self-doubt?

So, we feel doubt. And who the wants to feel that? So, intentional or not (likely not), we come up with a myriad of tricks to help us feel like we're good teachers, maybe even the best teachers. Problem is, there is a difference between feeling like a good teacher and being a good teacher.

In my opinion, it's often the ways we try to gloss over doubt and insecurity that get us into trouble. Not to spoil the ending but one major theme you're likely going to see throughout this book is the lengths we will go to in order to avoid feeling insecure about ourselves, or anything. This work in this book isn't about fixing our insecurities, not really. This is about becoming more aware of the ways we try to avoid them and, in the process, potentially deepen them.

Which brings us to the good stuff. Meaning the stuff we have all done to some degree but none are keen to admit to. I mean seriously, none of us are going to post our next Instagram pic with the caption, "Kombucha helps me feel my best while I manipulate people." If you do, please tag me.

Faking It: Manipulation and Tricking Ourselves into Feeling Legit

My Story: The Wannabe Guru

I only dipped my toe into wannabe gurudom, but, let me tell you, it felt gooooood. Like, imagine how double chocolate ice cream must feel (if it could feel) on a hot day when absolutely everybody wants some—that's how gurudom feels. I don't mean actually being a guru in the traditional sense, I mean being the appropriated stereotype of a guru commonly found in modern yoga settings. It's beyond feeling special. It's special on methamphetamines. And that wonderfully special and wanted-by-all feeling overran all my ethics and better judgement.

The first yoga class I ever taught was at an ashram in Rishikesh, India—*I know, how auspicious*. I was fresh out of my first yoga teacher training and, at the invitation of the Swami, was teaching a month-long session of karma (free) yoga. I wanted to be good at it. I wanted to be good at it so freaking bad. In my mind, I'd been one of the best students at the training and so my expectations of myself were high and mighty. However, there was one problem: I had next to no idea what I was doing. Any new yoga teacher is going to flail a little and I knew this but I reeeally didn't want that to be me. Otherwise, I might not be as special as I thought. So, I covered up my lack of knowledge and subsequent shame with what I have since come to call "Yoga Teacher Armour." Basically, I was super charming and pretended to be semi-enlightened. Only semi because I had just started teaching and wanted to remain somewhat humble.

It didn't take much to be a fake guru. Many people assume that as a yoga teacher we already have some sort of direct line to the universal truth. Taking it a step further into teaching like we do is easy. Acting like an omnipotent being that knows the secret of the cosmos came almost without thought or planning, it flowed in a way that was almost reflexive. I would say as little as possible and keep my answers to any questions vague but seemingly deep. I developed the habit of making meaningful, happy eye contact with everyone. I was distant from my students so they never really got to know me, but simultaneously talked about love and connection all the time. I showed vulnerability sometimes, but only when it served the purpose of making people like me more. Why did I do all this and how did I know to do it? Well, I'd watched other people who seemed enlightened act this way for years so it's what I did. The worst part is that as long as I could keep up the act, it worked. It worked really well.

In this, the most esoteric stage of my yoga journey, I taught a lot about chakras, healing sounds, and mantras. I was, at best, a novice in all these areas but found myself easily and almost effortlessly padding the edges of my knowledge with spiritual sounding flair. This "padding" can be done with anything, by the way, but it seems to happen more easily in energetic-based yoga practices. And, lord have mercy, did I go for it. The more I embellished, the more my predominantly Western students seemed to think I had some sort of special touch. After a while, I started believing I did too—take it from me that the line between faith in oneself and self-delusion is thinner than you might guess. I remember one guy asking me for a personalized sound to heal his throat chakra and I gave him one, intuitively. Maybe it worked for him and maybe it didn't, but that doesn't negate the fact that I, more or less, just made it up based on one month of study, some cool sounding jargon, and the belief that I was allowed to do this because I was me. One day, a couple of Western students ran into me on the street and bowed down to me. Okay, they bobbed a little in respectful greeting. But in my head, they were bowing before me, a manifestation of celestial bliss, who was showing them the path to freedom and love. I'm not exaggerating. Place a lost, insecure person in even a vague position of power and they will eat it up like meatless, non-dairy, gluten-free hamburgers.

Fake Always Falls Apart

This brings us to the conclusion of my pseudo-guru tale—I got sick. Well, in truth I had a bad experience with my novice Kundalini practice that left my nervous system in shaky tatters, but for the sake of brevity, let's call it sick (yes, I was most definitely teaching aspects of Kundalini Yoga when this happened and continued to do so after). Yoga teachers aren't supposed to get sick. We have super spiritual powers that protect us against that, don't we? I couldn't tell my students what was going on, it would have broken the façade that I'd worked so hard to create, so I tried to keep it going. I wasn't really conscious of this deception, I was just doing what I thought all yoga teachers were supposed to do and hoping that no one noticed. Eventually, inevitably, they did. Without my ethereal charms and feel-good pseudo-wisdom, class attendance dwindled and by the end of the month I was left with three semi-enthusiastic regulars whose attendance, I suspect, was based mostly on the class still being free. I was convinced that I'd failed my first test as a teacher: fake enlightenment. I also resented my students for not appreciating the amount of energy I had put into my performance. So, when I left the ashram I stopped teaching and practicing altogether until I felt I had the strength to once again, "fake it til I make it."

Manipulation vs Teaching

I think the greatest challenge to every modern day yogi is to differentiate between teaching and manipulating. Students will often unconsciously place teachers on pedestals as though we have all the answers, but that doesn't give us license to use that misconception to our own benefit, no matter how easy it is to do.

Part of living in society is having influence over other people and other people having influence over us. This give and take is part of healthy social interactions. Manipulation is influence that only flows in one direction and is primarily for the manipulator's benefit. When we are manipulating someone, we are pushing them to change their perceptions and/or behaviours through the use of mental and emotional trickery. Simply put, as a teacher, it's an end game of getting people to do what we want rather than helping them discern what's best for themselves. It's not about educating or empowerment, it's about us gaining and keeping control over other people. My yoga teacher armour felt so safe because it gave me unchallenged sway over everyone in the class.

The seeds of manipulative behaviours are usually sown when we were children attempting to get our emotional needs met. There's no shame in that—getting attention and affirmation at a young age is a matter of survival. Then we grow up and for some of us these behaviour patterns remain even though we no longer need them. There is much more that can be said about how and why we develop manipulative behaviours and what to do about it, but that is beyond the scope of the work we're doing here. There are ample resources out there if you want to do more research, just be sure to check the qualifications of whoever you learn from (yes, people can manipulate while apparently educating about manipulation).

The most common form of manipulation we see in yoga settings is charisma. I call it "manipulation light." It's a little dance we do with people to make them smile and feel good about themselves and, by way of that, us. It's a calculated self we show in order to be liked and get what we want (full classes, accolades, money, take your pick). It also makes people more likely to trust us and believe what we tell them is true. It can be as easy as always having a snappy quip to make others laugh or as calculated as remembering a detail about someone's personal life so we can bring it up later to show them we care.

As teachers, we all use charisma to varying degrees to engage the people in our classes. It's harmless fun when kept in check and not made the basis of our teaching methodology. Where charm starts to become dangerous is when we use it without self-awareness or boundaries and we let that ooey-gooey ice cream feeling overrun our better judgement. It's easy to say we'd never do that, but we all love attention, love people thinking we're the bees knees, and love our classes being full. Manipulation and charm are the easiest route to achieving all of these. I may not play guru anymore, but I still regularly check myself for relying on humorous charm in lieu of solid teaching.

Charisma, fake personas, and pseudo wisdom that plays to people's emotions to cover a lack of real content (also known as talking out of your ass) are just some ways manipulation can play out in yoga settings. Detecting manipulative behaviours in our own teaching can be tricky. It also takes a tremendous amount of courage. One telltale sign is that we like to hold ourselves as somehow above or separate from other people in the class/community and situations that might make us appear vulnerably human are something to be hidden or glossed over with spiritual rhetoric. Another sign is that as people progress in their practice they seem to become more dependent on us for answers instead of thinking for themselves. This dependent behaviour is common in students when, as teachers, we purposely hurt or stir up their emotions under the guise of teaching them something. This is sometimes called "truth telling" or "tough love." It's neither.

The truth of it is that many people are very unknowingly susceptible to being manipulated. It's happened to me many times in yoga/spiritual circles; it's not something to be ashamed of. People often come to yoga looking for something that is missing in their lives. An easy way to fill that existential hole is a person in a position of authority telling them they are a good person and that they belong. The point of their yoga then becomes less about their personal learning and practice, and more about changing to meet the teacher's expectations so that they can continue to belong. Let's just take a moment to reread that sentence, because it's a doozy. *The point of their yoga then becomes less about their personal learning and practice, and more about changing to meet the teacher's (our) expectations so that they can continue to belong.* People often mistake this conditional acceptance and subservience as a deep personal connection with the teacher. In truth this is the farthest thing there is from it—manipulation is the opposite of connection. Remember, healthy influence is supposed to go both ways. This dependency driven dynamic is why manipulation is so effective at filling up a room. Give a man a fish and he'll eat for a day, get a man to think he needs you in order to eat and you'll have him hooked on fish for life.

Spiritual Bypassing

It's hard not to want to be the teacher with all the answers, and the quickest route to feeling like that person is to fake it. Which brings us to spiritual bypassing. Also known as that thing other yoga people do, right?

Mastery of anything requires both theoretical and experiential knowledge (knowing stuff and then repeatedly trying to apply said stuff to real life situations). The premise is that we read or hear teachings that are meant to guide and inspire us; this is us gaining theoretical knowledge. We then take this theoretical knowledge and try putting it into practice and see what happens; this is how we gain experiential knowledge. In doing so we learn a whole lot more than the theoretical teaching alone could ever tell us. This real-life application of a theory is also known as praxis, if you want to get fancy. Teachings that give us a sense of where our spiritual road might lead are a double-edged sword. What can and often does happen is that our desire to progress can cause us to bypass experiential learning/praxis and go straight to an imagined endpoint based solely on theoretical knowledge. It's akin to our spiritual rubber never having met the road.

Spiritual bypassing is easy to judge and even easier to do. For many of us, it was how we were taught to practice and teach. Again, the easiest way to feel like a good teacher is to act the way we think a good yoga teacher would act; ethereal, calm, compassionate, detached, wise…(you know the picture). The problem with this approach is we haven't done enough of the prerequisite work required to genuinely achieve these states. We're just guessing at what they look/feel like based on an image—this is spiritual bypassing. And it's almost impossible to bypass without acting like a bit of a jerk. For instance, when a student says something like, "The way you teach doesn't respect my needs as a fat-bodied person," and the teacher replies with, "You need to let go of that ego-based identity, we're all one and the same," the teacher is using bypassing to avoid facing a valid critique. Another one from my own past is me telling a teacher," I'm just having a really hard time right now," and them responding with," That's only your mind's perception, you need to be more in your body and less in your head." See how that works? Using a spiritual bypass to shut down unwanted dialogue about all things uncomfortable, anyone?

To our greater detriment, all the confusion, failure, and ongoing effort of practice that we skip over when we bypass is the prerequisite work that ultimately qualifies us to teach. My favourite example is, "let it go." Letting go of something is an organic process that occurs as the result of our personal healing work (many many ways to go about this). Letting go as a stand-alone bypassing action is usually just well-intentioned denial. This is a great short-term solution for being a messy human but it gets us nowhere in the long run. The truth is that what we do not deal with adds up and will eventually start to weigh on us. If we do it as teachers, the weight of faking it can get very heavy indeed and manifest itself as bullying, disillusionment, imposter syndrome and a number of other problematic behaviours that we'll get to later.

I believe that this lack of experiential knowledge is why bypassing and manipulation are so often seen together—we use one to compensate for the other. It's a package that can sell well for a while, but, deep down, we know that sales depend on us keeping our charming guru armour on and never really being seen for who we are. That's a horrendous load to carry. Bypassing continues to be popular because many of us simply don't know better until we know better. We were taught bypassing as a spiritual endeavour by our teachers and so we went with it, unaware of the consequences.

I think, to an extent, bypassing is a natural phase of yoga. We start with high intellectual ideals and through time and practice this is cured into something more experientially based; this is called integration. Wise teaching requires integration, and integration is only possible when we take time to learn and practice without the immediate impulse to teach our initial assumptions. Wisdom isn't given, it's earned.

Using the "Exotic" to Feel Legit

This section is geared towards my fellow non-Indian yoga teachers. If you fall into this category and find yourself already coming up with counter arguments for whatever I might say here about using sacred practices from other cultures, let me say, "I know the feeling." If you fall into this category and find yourself already feeling smug because you see yourself as a woke ally to all peoples, let me say, "I know the feeling." If we're aiming to be open minded yoga teachers willing to look at truths that differ from our own, I recommend staying somewhere in between these two extreme positions—it requires a bit more thought but it's worth it.

A discussion around the roots of yoga and how to respect them while simultaneously allowing for innovation and evolution is a book in and of itself, and some really great books have been written on it. I'm not going to go into the finer points of what is and isn't cultural appropriation here; I'd rather give you links to teachers who have made this issue the focus of their work and let you learn from them (see the back of the book for suggestions). This referral to appropriate people/sources is what's commonly known as "staying in your lane" and we'll get into it in more detail in the section on professional boundaries. What I will share is my favourite definition of cultural appropriation: "Using the wisdom of elders without regard for their descendants" (original source unknown). Basically, utilizing the wisdom/practices/name of yoga (or any culture, religion, or philosophy) whilst consciously or unconsciously believing that we are somehow better than Indian people.

The issue with my early teaching persona wasn't so much that I was a white lady teaching an ancient Indian religion, it was that I was picking and choosing the parts of it I liked and doing whatever I wanted with them for personal gain. I got away with it because I was teaching people who knew even less about Hinduism and Yoga than I did. I did it because using the flashier aspects of Indian culture and Hinduism made me feel like a legit yogi. It's a lot like spiritual bypassing; I got the yogi feel without doing the experiential work and, in the process, missed the point. The problem was not with me, or with the content, but with my flippant approach to the content. Looking back, I was excited to belong to something meaningful, something with depth, and so I acted, dressed, and taught in a way that I thought signified my belonging. And while these signifiers worked on folks who didn't know better, they alienated and disrespected members of the very culture from which they were taken.

Another illustration of this behaviour is that after I stopped mantra as a personal practice, I continued to sing mantras at the end of my classes. I joked to friends that it was "insurance" in that, even if someone didn't like my class, my sweet voice singing to them in an ancient language would ensure they left thinking I knew my stuff. In retrospect, I often make jokes about things I'm not quite ready to admit yet. Seemingly 'exotic' spiritual practices can be like a trump card in that anyone who doesn't know better will usually assume we know how to use them and have earned the right to do so. That's how they are easily misused for manipulation and bypassing. This is one of the reasons why cultural appropriation is so offensive; it's not just borrowing the sacred, it's distorting it with an (possibly unconscious) ulterior motive. Again, I'm not saying your practice of yoga or any Indigenous spiritual tradition is by default appropriative, I'm saying get clear about why you're practicing this way and look for the impact this practice potentially has on the culture in which it originated.

As we move into the practices part of this section, I highly recommend two commitments here: 1) putting work into researching what cultural appropriation is, what it is not, and the multitude of issues that exist under this sometimes overused heading. By that I mean read up on multiple opinions and definitions that you both agree and disagree with and think about what you read. Like yoga, this isn't about finding a right answer, it's about shifting perspective. 2) Find a qualified guide/teacher to help you start doing the internal work of uncovering your personal biases, assumptions, stereotypes, etc. and feeling all the emotions that come with that. This second half is absolutely necessary in order for this information (theoretical) to become a shift in perspective (experiential). Without this second part, we are likely to fall into bypass-mode again and run the risk of becoming either closed-minded for the sake of personal comfort or using this new information as a points system we can use to feel superior to and police others with. Neither response does much good. Inclusion as a practice is addressed more thoroughly in the next section.

Your Story: Ever Faked it?

Do you or have you ever subscribed to the guru model (westernized or traditional) of teaching/learning yoga? Write about your experience (good, bad, anything). What is/was it like as a student and what is/was it like as a teacher?

What are your thoughts on the "fake it until you make it" strategy of teaching? Pros? Cons? Have you ever used a fake persona as a teacher? Was it yoga teacher armour or some other method? What were your motivations? To what degree was the persona problematic? To what degree was it beneficial?

Do you rely on charisma as a teacher? How much and in what situations do you depend on it more? Why do you think that is? Who are you without it?

Do you ever notice yourself "padding the edges" while teaching? When and how does it happen? Why do you think it happens?

Have you ever been manipulated by a teacher, or witnessed it happen to another person? How did you realize what was happening? How did that affect you?

What are your experiences with spiritual bypassing? Think about examples of theoretical and experiential learning from your own practice and the different impacts these two forms of learning have. If you can't think of any, keep an eye out for them in your practice.

Do you use sacred objects, language and/or practices from cultures other than your own when teaching? What is your purpose in doing so? How do you ensure you honour these practices, rather than simply appropriate and profit from them? What is your gut reaction to being asked to explain your motives?

What questions do you have about cultural appropriation? Are you willing to put in the time to research these questions to find answers for yourself? Why or why not? Be as honest with yourself as you can about your motives and explore their origins.

How does the idea of "gurudom" apply to newer trends in yoga such as self-help, life coaching, and movement science? How can manipulation and playing guru play out in these areas?

Any other aspects of faking it, manipulation, bypassing, appropriation you want to hash out? Go for it.

Practice Transparency and Praxis

Authenticity with Skill

After my attempt and subsequent failure at gururdom, I eventually returned to Canada and starting teaching again. Immediately my yoga teacher armour came back out. Why? Because I didn't know how else to teach. It's not that I thought teaching this way was wrong, it was that I thought I needed to get better at it. Shedding my wannabe guru addiction has been a slow, steady process that's taken years. It's hard not to want to believe that there is someone out there with all the answers. It's equally hard to not want to believe that person is me, even if I have to fake it get there. One of the best ways to do our part to dismantle this harmful culture in yoga is to stop pretending we are something we are not. Of course, this is easier said than done, which brings us to the practice of transparency.

Transparency is learning to skillfully be ourselves when we teach. Transparency doesn't require that we tell people everything about ourselves, just that we don't hide behind our yoga teacher armour or a fake persona. It is a way of protecting everyone involved from manipulation because it makes us clarify and account for ourselves as teachers. One of the most eye-opening experiences I have ever had as a yoga practitioner was realizing that it was not only okay for the people I taught to see me as human, but it made me a better teacher. And I mean really see me, as me. Not as a human on a higher plane of authentic existence and not as occasionally human when showing rehearsed vulnerability, but as a flawed real-life human with value and knowledge to share.

Here's a comparison of using vulnerability to manipulate versus using it to be transparent:

A teacher is telling a personal story about getting into a fight with their partner and how they used their inner yoga practice to help resolve it.

Manipulative: the story is curated to present the teacher as having maybe messed up a little, in a way that is more humorous than exposing, but ultimately prevails as the hero. Even in the midst of anger, they were able to be present and use their inner practice to resolve the conflict, ultimately strengthening the relationship. The moral of the story is that, with practice, it is possible for students to achieve the teacher's level of wisdom.

Transparent: the story is the story of the couple's fight, without elevation or embellishment. The teacher may or may not be the one to show presence and wisdom in the situation, maybe it was their partner or maybe it was neither of them in the moment. Perhaps wisdom came after the fact. The point of the story is illustrating the inner practice of yoga in a way that people can both relate to and apply in their own lives, not making the teacher look good.

Transparency is authenticity (yes, the dreaded A-word) done with discernment and self-awareness.

Praxis Before Practice

Let's come back to our dear friend praxis, also known as the process of experiential learning or the practical application of a theory. Probably the biggest challenge in achieving transparency is developing a deep awareness of our own processes, the processes we often skip when we bypass. Knowing how we learn, understand, and progress at yoga, and being able to articulate that as part of our teaching, is key for several reasons.

First off, it helps us better explain what the practice of yoga is. That is kind of a "duh" point but stop and really think about how easy it is to practice and teach something because we read somewhere that it was right, be it philosophy, self-help, or biomechanics. With a theoretical understanding we can tell people a right answer but we can't bring a teaching to life for them if we haven't tried living it ourselves. This is true for everything from forward bends to the Yamas and Niyamas. Whatever form of yoga we teach, we are going to be better at it if we understand and fully own our unique experience of it. This is not to say that our experience will be indicative of the experience of others, it most likely won't be, but knowing where we're at will help us meet others where they're at. Combining subjective experience (you could also call it "being real") with the broad strokes of theory—be it philosophy, anatomy or anything—is how we bring it all together and create genuine vibrancy in our teaching.

An example: As a brand new teacher, I could have taught from that perspective. I'm not saying I should have sat up at the front of the room and talked about how nervous I was and how little I knew. It's authenticity with skill, remember? Professional vulnerability in this case could have been me simply acknowledging that I was new, nervous, and yet still excited to teach and explore yoga with everyone. Without the added pressure of gurudom, my curiosity for the new material and my questions about everything could have fuelled the class and sparked excitement in my students. I know this because I have since tried it and simply telling a class I'm nervous is often the easiest way for everyone to stop feeling jittery and start to connect with one other. As it was, my suppression and bypassing of the experience left me exhausted and my students disinterested when I was no longer able to put on a good show for them.

Secondly, transparency gives the people we teach an example of what a yoga practice in progress looks like, which is far more powerful and supportive than giving them an image of some arbitrary endpoint. It is also far less likely to involve an appropriated stereotype of what we think that endpoint looks like. Teaching in this way takes away the pedestal and replaces it with a path that we walk down together. That sounds a bit sappy and it's meant to. Sharing the learning and growth of your yoga practice openly and honestly with each other is a beautifully sappy thing because it is a real connection—not a fake one built on emotional manipulation. Real connection to anyone requires a willingness to be vulnerable without agenda. As a teacher this can be as simple as disclosing that we don't practice asana everyday or admitting we don't know the answer to someone's question. The point in telling people isn't that we expect them to do anything about it, it's simply an acknowledgement of our human fallibility. It's being honest, and that in and of itself is freeing for everyone involved.

This brings us back to the discernment part of the transparency equation. We are who we are, unapologetically, but this does not mean it is all about us. We share what we share with the intent of showing our own practice and life as it has the potential to impact the people we teach. If an aspect of our life has nothing to do with what we are teaching, then there may not be a need to share it. An example: talking about a recent fight with our partner at the beginning of an online class because we are upset, alone at home, and want to talk about it is overstepping. What we could do instead is acknowledge to the class that we are not having a good day and seek emotional support from someone in our personal life (we'll get more into boundaries later). If we are comfortable after the dispute has been settled, we could share the process with the class as part of a lesson if we think it would benefit them and we feel okay about it (the key being that it benefits them, not just us). We are however we are on any given day, and that is absolutely fine, but we don't need to make it all about us.

Your Practice: How Will You Bring Transparency and Praxis into Your Teaching

Describe transparency in a way that works for you. How can you cultivate transparency in your life? What might it look/feel like in your teaching? What challenges do you foresee with being more transparent? What benefits?

Can you think of teachers you've had in the past that were transparent? How did it feel being in their classes? How did their honesty help you learn? How did it encourage your praxis?

For the following three categories, list some real-life personal experiences that have come up while teaching or that have affected you as a teacher (example given). Then write out ways you could practice transparency about these experiences while in the role of teacher (you may choose not to talk about it but still not actively hide it).

Your Personal Practice:

Example: A old injury acting up.

Your Teaching:

Example: Someone asks you a question you don't entirely know the answer to.

Your Personal Life:

Example: You come to class in an awful mood.

How can you tell the difference between manipulation and transparency? In your own actions and in the actions of others?

How can transparency and praxis help you stay grounded? What does that look like for you? What does it change?

How can transparency help diminish cultural appropriation in your yoga practice? Think about being honest about who you are rather than projecting an appropriative image of who you want to be. How does appreciating rather than appropriating help clarify the unique gifts YOU bring to yoga? (Susanna Barkataki, 2021)

How does praxis apply to your style of practice and teaching? What does it look like? How does it feel? What are the benefits and what are the challenges?

How can praxis take the place of spiritual bypassing in your practice? How does it feel to know you don't need to have all the answers or pretend to? How does this change the goal of your practice and teaching?

Super Special Me: Selfishness and Exclusivity

My Story: Follow My Bliss

" Special Me" teaching is most definitely a thing. And this one also feels reeeeeeeally good. It's like being the star of your own reality show—but it's your yoga class. It's coming into the classroom with a bravado and confidence that comes from thinking you are the absolute spiritual shit. The third yoga teacher training I did (I'm not naming names because it doesn't matter) was high octane special yogi all the way. I don't think that's what the teacher intended for me to get out of it—I think she was shooting for empowerment—but what I took away was that the most important person in the classroom was me. What I wanted to teach and how I wanted to go about teaching it was what mattered.

I didn't wake up one morning and decide, "Screw the students, this is the Tori Show." Narcissistic tendencies snuck in and I mistook them for confidence and the natural progression of an introspective practice. Whoops.

Some obvious telltale signs of "Special Me" teaching include teaching/demoing poses that no one in the class can do (think teaching as a spectator sport), doing involuntary acro yoga on students and calling it "adjustments", long-winded talks on philosophy and life advice that no one asked for, and no one ever disagreeing with or challenging you in class. Some less obvious signs include everyone in your classes seeming similar to you in body/lifestyle/culture/beliefs, a strong desire to be seen as inspirational, and not wanting to engage in learning that challenges your belief system or view of yourself. As a side note, it's really easy to slide into a self-focused teaching style when we're teaching online classes because we're most likely in a room by ourselves with minimal to no feedback from others.

My full on "Special Me" stage lasted about a year. It was fun. Most of my classes at this time were more or less the same style (teaching was about what I wanted to do, remember), a fast-paced flow style of class with minimal time spent explaining modifications or using props. Keeping the dancer-like flow going was what mattered most. My regular students loved it—because the only students who stuck around from week to week were the ones who could do it. One day, into this Tori show came an older lady, who told me she had both yoga experience and chronic back pain. After this initial conversation I honestly don't remember even looking in her direction for the rest of the class. What I do remember is that I really didn't care about her, her experience of the class, or if she got anything out of it because she wasn't my style of yogi.

I may not remember her during that class but I remember exactly how I felt when I found out who she was a week later. She was a senior Iyengar teacher. Like, senior teacher in the sense that she had taught my favourite teachers and I'd heard about her for years but never met her. This lady knew things about bodies and yoga that I didn't even know existed. Her not telling me who she was, I think, had been a humble kindness on her part. I only found out who she was later because one of my teachers told me. This senior teacher had said nothing to my teacher about my class, just that she'd tried it. Again, a kindness on her part. She never tried it again. Sometimes it's enough of a wake-up call to simply know someone has seen our bullshit; they don't need to call us on it. It was a harsh realization that, while I'd been a great teacher to some, I'd been a terrible teacher to many. Acknowledging this embarrassing truth knocked me right off my pedestal and onto my apparently not-so-special ass.

The Trouble with Inspiring People

Turns out that what I thought was confidence was actually arrogance. Nobody ever tells you how good arrogance feels when you're caught up in it. If wannabe gurudom is feeling like you're ice cream on a hot day, then arrogance is thinking you're ice cream on hot day when in actuality it's the dead of winter. The reason "special me" teaching feels so empowering is because we don't leave any room for questions or doubt. Mainly because we don't leave any room for people who would cause us to question, or doubt what we are doing. You can tell the difference between real confidence and arrogance because the former leaves room for others; the latter never does.

The people who would potentially challenge us come to one class and don't fit in; we never see them again and quickly forget them. Those who remain fit into our mold so well that they excel and we then interpret their progress as a testament to our teaching ability. In reality, they were just similar to us to begin with. It's my belief that this is what's commonly referred to as "inspiring people", and inspiring people is not the same as teaching.

The trouble with wanting to inspire people is that we inevitably hold them to our own subjective standards and vice versa. We inspire people who are already like us to be more like us and their emulation further entrenches our belief that we are right. It bolsters that "special me" feeling through a feedback loop of everyone agreeing with each other because we're all alike. We all feel nice but no one learns anything. We get called a great teacher not because we are, but because people will praise us to no end for reaffirming what they already want to believe is true. It's easy to feel enlightened when no one ever asks you to explain yourself. This is how yoga cliques can delude us into thinking our preferences are wisdom and our opinions are truths. Exclusivity deprives everyone of real growth.

Now, if you've been teaching for a while then you know that there is no such thing as a one-size-fits-all-class. Trying to accommodate everyone often means we end up accommodating no one—yoga classes occur within a broad spectrum for a reason. We also can't please everyone who happens to wander into our class, nor should we try. Some people will not like our teaching regardless of how we go about it and there is no such thing as a class that is for absolutely everyone. If you love teaching a very specific type of class, that's absolutely fine. The question is how do we view, and subsequently respond, to the person who shows up and doesn't fit into our lesson plan? Those people who not only challenge our inspirational mold, but ask us to potentially change it? There's no definitive right answer to this question, it's one of those sit-and-ponder-it, experiential learning, praxis-type situations. A vinyasa teacher walks into a class to sub Yoga for Back Pain, what do they do?

If you're reading this and nodding along because you're thinking of all the other teachers who do this, you're missing the point. We all do it, or have the capacity to, to some degree. I'm tempted to do it right now because I'm so special as to be writing about it (insert eye-roll emoji). The easiest way to feel like we are included in something special is to exclude others in some way—even if it's over their own exclusivity. This doesn't mean we aren't allowed to have opinions, disagree with each other, or hang out with people similar to us; it means not using this to bolster our own ego (yes, I mentioned the e-word). Fun example: One of my favourite teaching shirts has the word "decolonize" on it. A guy who once, and only once, showed up for a class was dumbfounded as to what this meant. I explained but the whole time I was silently judging him. I thought I hid it, but nope, my distaste showed. I had the opportunity to connect with someone and potentially make a real difference and instead I chose to be a snob about it. In doing so, I lost the opportunity and the student. I don't blame him for never coming back.

Social Media

None of this sound familiar? Think of your social media presence. We get a group of followers who are likely similar to us and agree with most of what we have to say and how we choose to practice. There's your "special me" feedback loop, also known as cognitive bias. To put a new spin on an old yoga scene favourite, "Your vibe attracts...people who agree with you."

For marketing purposes this "reality TV star" approach works really well. Marketing shows people an image that they want to emulate and/or be a part of in hopes that they will literally "buy in." If we do it well, it works. As much as I would love to tell you yoga is a meritocracy, where those with the greatest skill rise to the top, this just is not the case. For most of us, marketing is a necessary part of modern day teaching and getting good at it is nothing to be ashamed of. The point I am making with bringing it up is that's dangerous to confuse successful marketing with good teaching; they are two completely different agendas and skill sets, or, at least in my opinion, they should be. Teaching in the same way we would market ourselves is narcissistic teaching.

Personally, some of my most successful posts have simply been well articulated one-sided opinions that my followers agreed with. It was fun, felt good, and it got my name out there, but it wasn't teaching. A similar situation in a class setting could be teaching a sequence online that makes me feel great. I spend the class talking about how and why this sequence makes me feel great without ever focusing on variations to help students figure out how to make it feel great for them. When we are marketing, we want people to pay attention to us. When we are teaching, we want people to be paying attention to themselves.

Your Story: Have You Been Special Lately?

What are your thoughts and experiences with "special me" thinking? When is it problematic and when is it not? Where is the line for you between confidence and arrogance?

Have you ever been more focused on yourself than the people you are teaching? Why and how did it play out? How did it feel? Did your self focus cause harm to others? Be accountable but don't be too hard on yourself.

Do you want to be seen by others as inspirational and/or a leader? Why? What need does this fulfil for you? Is this need a higher priority than the people you wish to lead/inspire? If the answer is yes, or occasionally yes, what affect does this have on your teaching? Positive and negative.

How do you tell the difference between feeling like a great yoga teaching and acting like a great yoga teacher?

Who are your classes for? How and why?

Have you ever taken a class where you felt you weren't welcome or didn't belong? How did it feel? What did the teacher(s) do that made you feel unwelcome? If you haven't, write about why you think you have never experienced this and the potential blind-spots that has created in your teaching.

Are all of your yoga students similar to you in age, class, culture, gender, and ability? What effect might this have on your teaching, your view of yoga, and how you view yourself? If you don't know if your students are similar to/different than you, why haven't you noticed?

How do you approach people who potentially have different needs than others in a class? What assumptions do you make? How do you approach people who don't do (for whatever reason) what you want to teach in a class?

Do you sometimes gauge your worth/ability as a teacher by your social media presence? What are the pros and cons of that? How can it influence how you act while teaching?

What cliques and feedback loops exist in your life? How do these closed circles affect you and your perception of the world? How do you respond to outside perspectives and opinions?

What other thoughts, feelings, stories do you have on this topic?

Practice Humility and Inclusion

Why Special Sucks

Okay, so we all have the special tendency. It feels pretty great for us and for those who are similar to us—everyone in the clique is happy so really, where's the problem? Well, here's an almost identical story:

Shorty before my run in with the senior teacher, another woman came to a few classes who didn't fit my mold. She wasn't a very social person and kept largely to herself except for when asking me questions about what I was teaching, questions I answered but did not appreciate. One day I decided to adjust her pelvis in child's pose without asking her (I never asked in those days). The adjustment went fine, from my perspective, until I let go and she sat up and, for the whole class to hear, said, "Tori, maybe you should ask people before you touch them instead of coming up from behind and surprising them." I was shocked by her statement, but ignored her and kept teaching, so as to not disrupt the flow of the class, or that's what I told myself. After class, when she had left, my regulars stayed behind to support me and reaffirm I was a great teacher by telling me, "She's just difficult." She never came to another class and, apart from my own hurt feelings, I never thought of her again until years later when I started learning about trauma sensitive yoga and how adjustments can trigger people into fight/flight/freeze responses (see the resource section for more information on trauma sensitive yoga). In light of that information, I was 100% in the wrong.

The big difference between these two stories is that at the time, the senior teacher's opinion mattered to me and the "difficult" woman's opinion did not. I was only open to learning the lesson when it came from someone who I deemed important. Exclusivity is like putting on educational blinders; if we only learn from those we deem "special" enough to teach us, we are going to miss out on 90% of life's lessons. Subsequently, we're not going to grow very much as people or teachers (to tie this into the previous section, lack of growth usually leads to theoretical, bypass-laden teaching).

My other point in telling you this second story is to dispel the myth that, "those people aren't in this class." For starters, who exactly are "those" people? Do we mean people who have life experiences and needs that differ from our own? Based on the assumptions in the standard Western yoga class model this could include people dealing with trauma, mental illness, chronic pain or injury, eating disorders, and addictions, as well as people who are LGBTQIA2s+, have a skin colour that isn't white/light, are above a size 12, are seniors, aren't middle or upper class, grew up and/or live in a different culture from us, navigate personal and structural racism on a daily basis, are the targets of fat-phobia, have visible or hidden disabilities, and the list could go on. That is a whole lot of people to never ever be in one of our classes. Chances are, people different from our yoga norm have been in our classes all along, we just didn't see them.

Changing Your Attitude, Change Your Teaching

Inclusion can be tricky because it flies in the face of how so many of us were taught to teach. We can't be experts on inclusion because you can't be an expert on someone else's experience. When we take the expert approach we run the risk of becoming the "woke" person in the room who knows what's best for everyone but doesn't connect with anyone. Inclusion is not about having the right answers. For this reason, I encourage you think about inclusion not as a checklist that we get right, but as an attitude we bring to every situation. In this way, we can bring inclusion into whatever style of yoga we choose to teach. Yes, some things might change in our approach, but we don't have to throw the baby out with a bathwater. We can love our yoga without making it solely about us.

As I said earlier, it's impossible to cater to absolutely every person who wanders into a class; teaching group classes is, out of necessity, done in broad strokes rather than person-specific details. If it's an online class, the strokes are even more broad because we most likely don't even know who it is we're teaching. However, there has to be a line where we accept responsibility for those who walk through our door or click on our link. We need to acknowledge both who is the class with us while also noticing who is consistently absent. If everyone in our classes happens to be similar to us, chances are we that we are excluding people. Please note, this is not the same as intentionally creating a safe space specifically for people who are excluded from other, more generalized spaces. Chances are, anyone who has felt a need for this kind of safe space is already more aware of the issues surrounding inclusion and diversity in yoga than someone who has never personally been affected.

The key to teaching inclusive yoga is, in my opinion, humility. It's realizing that not everything is about us, for us, or known by us. This is easier agreed with than done. Just as arrogance is often confused with confidence, I think insecurity is often confused with humility. Insecurity comes from doubting ourselves and believing we are less than others (more on that later), while real humility is not seeking to put ourselves above others (which we tend to do in order to avoid feeling insecure). Without humility there cannot be inclusion. Humility creates an openness to learn, change, and challenge because we are not concerned with maintaining our "special" status. Unity isn't everyone agreeing with us, it's learning to engage with, respect, and appreciate our differences. Real humility is undervalued and undersold; possibly because it doesn't mix well with social media, but, as I said earlier, marketing and teaching are two different skills.

Putting That Attitude Into Practice

I know a lot about trauma because I have experienced my fair share and know how it can be either triggered or soothed by yoga. It turns out I hate adjustments just as much as the "difficult" woman in my story, I just never realized it because I would freeze and disassociate when touched unexpectedly during class. Oddly enough, this made me seem like the perfect malleable student until I began healing— that's when I became the difficult student telling teachers to go away and not touch me. While my personal experience can help me to cultivate empathy for others who similarly find themselves at odds with common yoga norms, it does not make me an expert or a spokesperson for anyone else's needs and wants. I have no idea what it feels like to be a Black person with societal-based trauma entering a yoga classroom full of white people. I have no idea what goes through a non-binary person's heart and mind when they walk through the doors of a yoga studio and only see two change room signs. I don't know the frustration of being in a wheelchair and trying to find a studio with physical accessibility. This may seem obvious, but it is a very slippery slope from wanting to know more about inclusivity to trying to make ourselves out to be an authority on it and other people. Specialness is insidious like that.

In light of that, I'm not going to give you a list of inclusive practices. I can't. Doing so would be me trying to be an expert on something I can never be an expert on. It would also be me taking credit for the work of the people who have taught me (specialness is so very insidious). Instead, I'm sending you to the source by providing a whole list of teachers and educators. Each with their own unique experiences, insights, wisdom, and approach to changing and broadening what we see as being "normal." Many of them are people I continue to learn from myself.

I honestly think the best way to learn about people's differing experiences in yoga, and life, is to spend a bit of time each week scrolling through a hashtag you'd never use on social media—preferably one that makes you a bit uncomfortable and/or that you can't personally relate to (a few examples could be #transisbeautiful #bodypositive #blackgirlmagic). Don't scroll to figure anyone out, just read what people have to say with an open mind and see where it takes you. Follow some of these new people to diversify the voices in your feed. Consider buying their trainings and services instead of who you would usually learn from in order to expand your yoga circle and increase your awareness of the world around you.

Again, humility is key and humility is not the same as self-doubt or playing small. It takes courage to talk to someone about the derogatory comment they made about Muslim people before class. Especially if we don't see anyone we could easily categorize as Muslim in our studio. Commitment to inclusion takes balls.

We do not need to be experts, all it takes is a commitment to learning and doing better for those in front of us. Doing the personal work of continuously unpacking our biases and noticing blind spots is step one. ("I never realized someone might find _____ difficult/offensive/triggering/scary but I do now so I'm going to _____.") Continuing to do this work with humility so as to not use this new awareness to feed into "special me" mentality is step two. Both are ongoing and both pair very nicely with transparency. The best thing we can do for any person in our class is not make their experience about us.

Practical information on how to foster inclusive yoga spaces along with recommendations for educators are included in the "People To Follow and Learn From" section.

Your Practice: How to Bring Humility and Inclusion into Your Teaching

What does teaching for both you AND your students feel/look like?

What is the difference between insecurity and humility? What do both feel like in your body? How does one act in comparison to the other? What does real confidence as a teacher feel like for you?

How do you want to interact with and impact people who come to your classes? How can these interactions be less about you and more about them? How can confidence help you be inclusive in these situations?

List all the classes you teach. Who are they for and is that reflected in what you are teaching? Are there changes that need to be made so that the class better fits the students? If all your classes and students are the same, would you consider branching out? Why or why not? How can you branch out without slipping into special me territory?

What potential challenges do you see with practicing humility while still marketing yourself and your classes? How can you find the balance?

Looking back, has your yoga excluded others? How and why? What were/are the consequences of this? What barriers exist that could exclude people from your classes? Are these things within your power to change? How can you change/lessen these barriers?

What do you think the term 'cultural humility' means? How can you practice it, especially if you are part of the dominant culture where you live? How does this tie into creating an attitude of inclusion in your teaching?

Are there aspects of yoga that change when you view them with an inclusive attitude? What might this change in how you approach teaching them? Don't worry about a right answer, this is about practicing a different way of thinking. (Praxis, baby!)

How can "special me" thinking derail an inclusive attitude? How can you support inclusion and inclusive practices without taking students/business away from marginalized educators and/or stealing their ideas and words?

Inclusion is an attitude, backed up by action. What are you going to do to continue to keep taking your blinders off? Please be specific.

Owning Too Much Power:
Authority and Dogma

My Story: No One Expects the Yoga Inquisition

Oh Lord, this one's rough.

I went through this mighty and all knowing teacher stage after my fifth yoga related training—are you getting that the amount of trainings someone has doesn't mean they necessarily know how to teach and/or they don't still have blind spots? Good.

I was certain I had figured this whole yoga thing out. Again, I'm not going to name the training, but it was one that was very precise in terms of alignment and sequencing and was backed up with a lot of great research. I liked it so much I did it twice. The knowledge was grand, but it was aggravating at the same time because almost everyone else hadn't figured these amazing truths out yet (aggravating in that wonderful way that is deeply satisfying because it allowed me to feel superior to others). I wanted people to acknowledge and respect the brilliance I had earned and I aimed to get it from them because I felt I deserved it. Self-righteousness is a real bitch, especially when we're absolutely positive that we're right.

This period was also after my second month-long intensive with an Adviata Vedanta (non-dualist philosophy) teacher in India. Basically, I was in full existential born-again mode. As often as my wonderfully harsh teacher had told me, "This is not about getting a right answer you can take a picture of and put in your spiritual scrapbook. Don't be a tourist," I most definitely had a picture and I was showing it off to everyone. "Look at me! I have the answer to existence, and you don't because your practice is stupid." It wasn't always that bad...but it was sometimes that bad. Again, we are all easily dreadful when we're sure we're in the right.

Both sets of knowledge were a relief in the way that concrete right/wrong answers usually are. I had the correct rules for yoga and I had the correct rules for existence, what more could a yogi want? This is always the appeal of dogma—it gives us clear and easy rules to follow in order to be good. It also provides us with the duality to classify anything that doesn't fit those rules as bad. The result was my teaching style became a little like a yoga version of the Spanish Inquisition.

It snuck into my classes in subtle ways and then slowly grew and festered into something decidedly not love and light. A person would begin to share an insight they'd had, and I wouldn't bother to listen because I really didn't care about their infantile practice. Someone would request an exercise in class I didn't approve of, and I'd either turn it into a joke at their expense or over explain why what they wanted to do was terrible. A student wouldn't do what I said and rather than respecting their choice I'd explain to the entire class the importance of why what I wanted them to do was important, shaming the rogue student in the process. If someone came up with an alternate theory or a question, rather than discussing it with them, I'd usually just shoot them down. Everything became about my having the right answers, which is another way of saying everything became about establishing my expertise and protecting my authority. As always, I didn't see it this way at the time, in my eyes I was showing people tough love and the truth. I couldn't see that my tough love was dominance and my truth was highly subjective. If I had to pick a low point in my teaching career, this would be it.

Call it what it is and own it: Bullying

Authoritative and fear-based teaching comes in many guises—tough love, speaking truth, owning our power, showing people their shadow, confidence (we mistake a lot of things for confidence)—but what it is, in my opinion, is bullying. Maybe stop and take a deep breath here if you realize that this has been you. It's a hard one to admit. Be accountable, but also, be kind to yourself. Again, we don't know better until we know better.

Authority is a tricky thing to navigate. Especially when we are so sure that what we are doing is right (I know, I have said that multiple times already, but it's so key). I mentioned social work's troublesome past at the beginning of the book. That past, which in Canada included taking Indigenous children away from their parents and causing widespread generational trauma in the process (known as the 60s Scoop and worth googling), was built on the foundation of authority and believing, "I know what's best for you even if you don't agree with me."

We get very few models in life for how to handle positions of authority well and we get even fewer pointers on how to be in these positions ourselves without making them an outlet for our own personal needs. It's not always as obvious as calling someone out during class. It can be as subtle as how our treatment of someone changes after they disagree with us on something, don't do what we think is best for them, or, Lord forbid, love a style of yoga that we think is sub-par.

The hardest work for me as teacher has been owning the potential within myself to misuse the authority granted to me when I stand at the front of a class. It's easy to look at celebrity teachers who have fallen from grace as an anomaly. It's comforting to see them as people who lost their way, who didn't "deal with their shit", or as outright villains. I can only speak for myself, but I know that part of the reason I want to "other" these teachers so badly is because of what they reflect back to me. They point to my own potential to be a pompous jerk. I have had a lot of great teachers in my life, but I also have learned from some bullies. In most cases, I didn't realize this dynamic until years after the fact, long after I'd adopted some of their tactics as my own.

Bullying is not a character trait we are born with, it's a learned behaviour (National Association of School Psychologists, 2003). Why and how we get hooked by holding power over another person is different for each of us—I can't tell you why bullying may take root in you, but I can share insights on my own experience. Bullies and victims are not a strict dichotomy—we can be bullied as children and wind-up bullying others later in life (Haltigan and Vaillancourt, 2014). That's me. I was bullied throughout elementary school—I was a dirt covered, heathen-esque tomboy in a small country school full of pure and proper Christian girls. While I believed I had dealt with the hurt and repercussions of that experience long before I started teaching yoga (I wrote whole papers on it while studying to be a social worker), it resurfaced in ways I never expected the moment I stepped up to lead a class full of pure and proper yogic women.

Bullying, for me, was unconsciously using that which hurt me early in life to try and protect myself from that hurt ever happening again. Even when the situation was entirely different, and I was in no real danger. As a teacher, bullying, like manipulation, helped me feel safe because dominating others made me feel in control. Combine that with an unquestionable doctrine of how to practice yoga and I felt invincible. It made me feel snug as a bug in a dogmatic rug. Everyone deserves to feel safe but not when it comes at someone else's expense. Make no mistake, when we make authority the cornerstone of our teaching, people are going to get hurt.

As teachers, because of the sway we have over our students, we need to be especially mindful of where/when we feel unsafe and how we might compensate for that while teaching. I'm sure you're noticing by now, doing what makes us feel good does not always align with good teaching. Like wannabe gurudom or specialness, domination can be intoxicating.

Dogma Doesn't Work

As much as it's become en vogue to dismiss yoga dogma, it's much harder to break our inclination towards strict right/wrong answers. Like spiritual bypassing, while it's easy to point out dogmatic beliefs in other people's practices, it's much harder to turn that same critical eye on ourselves and what we believe to be true. In my case, reality stepped in and didn't give me much of a choice.

Professionally, my authoritative stance was challenged when new research started emerging on how the body works and moves. According to most of this research, my expertise was either misguided or outright wrong. In addition, I had a workaholic-induced breakdown and realized that no amount of ancient non-dualist philosophy was going to heal the effect of trauma on my nervous system or subsequent maladaptive coping mechanisms. So, I got over my all-knowing self and started going to therapy.

Both the style of yoga I taught and Advaita philosophy had/have merit. I still incorporate both into in my teaching and daily life, but I no longer hold either as ultimate, universal truths because, as nice as that would be, they're not. These are simply what works for me, usually. Nothing conceptualized or practiced by humans is going to be true for all humans. If you've checked out some of the resources on inclusion I'm sure you're already getting a sense of just how different we all are. Even if we are all one, as my chosen philosophy states, we do not all need or want the same things and none of us is capable of deciding what is or is not true for another person. The Buddha may have been a brilliant exception, but he's not the rule. And even he sucked at teaching people when he first started out. Personally, I like to remind myself occasionally that this year's cure-all is next year's "Anusara who?" It helps me take everything I learn with a grain of salt and stay off my high horse.

And again, therapy. There are things I can show you in this book and things I can help you understand and articulate better but healing those old hurts is beyond me. If you get the sense you have the inclination towards being a bully, or feel deeply triggered by anything in this book, I suggest reaching out to someone who can support you, personally and/or professionally.

Your Story: How Do You Handle Authority?

Have you ever taught something you were absolutely sure was right? How did that self assurance feel and how did it influence you as a teacher? How did it affect your ability to see, hear, and respond to others? Positive and negative.

How does having power over someone else make you feel? Have you ever been a bully? How did it feel? How do you feel in hindsight?

What are your thoughts on dogma? Does it help you or hinder you as a teacher? Do you like and possibly cling to clear right/wrong answers? (no right/wrong answer to this)

Have you ever been bullied? How did you react and how did it feel? What were the long term consequences, if any?

Are you someone who society deems as having more or less authority? How can this affect you as a student? How can it affect you as a teacher?

As a student, what positive and negative role models have you had for navigating authority and power?

What's your reaction to feeling vulnerable while you are teaching? What's your reaction to vulnerability in others while you are teaching? Do you see vulnerability as a strength, a weakness, or a bit of both? Why?

What is your emotional reaction to someone in class saying "no" to you or not doing what you want? (NO WRONG ANSWER) What's your initial reaction? What's your ideal response?

What other thoughts, feelings, stories do you have on authority and dogma?

Practice Empathy and Autonomy

Create a "No" Friendly Environment

A breaking point for me with dogma and authority was the disembodied look in one student's eyes after I hoisted her up into a handstand she did not want to do. I felt justified at the time because it was done in the name of me helping her face her fears. Fears that I had decided she had and that I had decided it was time for her to face. She had opted not follow suit with the rest of class and I had called her out in front of everyone and made her go up. I knew she had the physical ability to do it so making her go up seemed the obvious "empowered teacher who empowers others" choice. Four months later I ran into her on the street and discovered she was seven months pregnant and so not going upside down for fear of harming her baby; something I hadn't even considered in my expert analysis of what was best for her.

That she didn't say "no" to me during that class is not so much her fault as it is mine. Most of us get conditioned to roll over for authority and I had created an environment in that class that made saying no to me extremely difficult. She likely went along with what I wanted because that is what we are taught to do with authority figures. In that moment her practice was no longer her own, I'd taken it away for the sake of my misinformed know-how. In retrospect, her disembodied state after was one I recognized from my own practice. I'd been pushed and prodded by my teachers (some, not all) and so I pushed and prodded my own students in the same way, all in the name of being a strong teacher. This is one way abusive teaching cycles continue.

No one likes rejection, in any situation. I know the surge of shame it can bring when a person rejects the help I want to offer them. I also know how easy it is to mask that shame by turning it into blame directed at the student and label them as "problematic" or "not open." Thing is, when we are in the role of teacher we are obligated to be better than our protective childhood impulses. That is why it is so important that we don't bypass any part of who we are in order to appear like better teachers. What we refuse to acknowledge about ourselves has a way of affecting everyone around us, especially those we teach. This dark side we all have is sometimes referred to as our "shadow side" though that term has become a bit romanticized in my opinion. Romanticizing can be a slippery slope towards bypassing. In reality, our shameful bits just are what they are, and they are not something that ever entirely goes away. The best we can do in addition to our own personal work is to create environments that minimize the potential for our shadowy bits to harm others.

How we break down abusive teaching is by creating environments where people can disagree with us without repercussions. Truth is, that even if what we want for someone is bang-on what they need, it does not give us the right to disregard their opinion on the matter. When we do, it creates an environment that disempowers everyone in the room but us. This is a dynamic that severely limits everyone else's potential as well as our own ability to feel empathy. Think about it—when we don't consider someone's experience or knowledge as equally valid to our own, it's very easy not to care about it, or them. This lack of responsiveness is what makes teaching dogmatically so easily de-humanizing. In short, we start to care about yoga more than we care about the people we are teaching it to.

Empathy and Autonomy

A few years ago I decided to make my teaching motto, "I care about people more than I care about yoga." It's my way of reminding myself to practice empathy and autonomy when I'm at the head of a class. Autonomy and empathy are a bit of a chicken and the egg situation—it doesn't really matter which comes first but developing one will naturally help us develop the other.

Autonomy means that everyone in a class is recognized as having the right to self-direction, also known as self-determination or agency.

Empathy is seeing the inherent worth in everyone and valuing their unique life experiences, even if we can't personally relate to those experiences. That last bit is important; we don't have to share in someone's experience in order to empathize with them. So, if we choose to practice empathy in our teaching, we naturally grow to value autonomy as a means of honouring everyone's unique needs and experiences. This does not mean we don't have anything to teach people, but that we care more about the person than we care about what we want to teach said person. It's a matter of getting our priorities straight.

An example: I still teach handstands in some of my classes. We lead up to them throughout class so that by the end everyone has worked with all the elements of doing a handstand but not the whole; I tell them as much. I usually give four options 1) work on handstand, 2) work on handstand with my help (for in-person classes) or with props I've shown them how to use (in-person or online), 3) work on refining one of the elements I previously taught instead of the whole, or 4) do legs up the wall or something else that better suits your needs today. This provides structure and guidance while also allowing space for choice (autonomy). If someone doesn't feel confident in making that choice on their own, I can use my knowledge to help them decide, but I don't get the final say. In person, this can be done through asking questions and having a discussion. Online, we can provide variations while encouraging everyone to do what they feel is best for them on that day (empathy). This mindset as a teacher is another way of understanding empowerment, shared empowerment that is. We are powerful, kick-ass beings with something great to share and *so is everyone else in the room with us.* Real personal power does not come at anyone else's expense.

But what about when it's necessary to push people in order for them to get better? Maybe you're asking that, maybe you're not. Regardless, my answer is that it's never necessary. What sounds more motivating to you personally: a teacher pushing you to do more because you need to become stronger or a teacher cheering you on for the strength you already have? They both might yield the same results, but one shames while the other uplifts.

De-centring Instead of Dominating

While always having the right answers promotes dependency, the ability to acknowledge what we do and don't know promotes honest communication and trust. We help people trust themselves when we care about their experience and support their ability to choose what is best for them. People learn to surrender to their yoga practice, not surrender to us. As we build this mindset into our teaching, we start to create a community where we may be the catalyst but we are not the centre. I'll add that, while authority and dogma feel good, they can't compare to the feeling of honest human connection and community.

Which brings us to one of my absolute favourite teaching ideals, an alternate, but complementary, explanation of the term praxis. Praxis can also mean that since we all share in this continual experience of learning/relearning; we are all simultaneously both teachers and students, all mixed together and helping each other on the way to liberation (Freire, 1968). Please reread that gem as many times as you like. Basically, we're all in it together and on the same level. In a yoga class, we are temporarily in the role of teacher and someone else is in the role of student. In another situation, those roles would be reversed. Our expertise is impermanent and situational, just like everything else in life. It's quite yoga-ish, isn't it? If you really let the idea of praxis sink in, it's a huge relief. We are not isolated in our attempts to walk the walk of what we are learning, others are beside us the entire way. We are not just some lone teacher with right answers, we are a part of a collection of people all learning and relearning from each other for our collective benefit and shared liberation. We can't know absolutely everything and the good news is we don't have to. Expertise is a communal practice.

Your Practice: How Will You Bring Empathy and Autonomy into Your Teaching

Think back on a time when a student disagreed with you or didn't do what you thought they should. Try to view that situation through the lens of empathy (you understand what they feel) and autonomy (you respect their right to choose). Does viewing the situation and person in this manner change your response? If what the students wants to do is potentially dangerous, what do you do then?

If you belong to a yoga lineage or specific school how will you balance honouring tradition with upholding personal autonomy? How can you maintain and protect traditional wisdom without sliding into dogmatic views? If you are not part of a lineage, speak to whatever you tend to get dogmatic about (movement science, anyone?).

Give examples of how to teach the following with empathy and autonomy. Again, it's not about a right answer, it's about getting creative with how to apply new skills.

Inversions:

Adjustments:

Savasana:

Class opening:

Seated forward bends:

Pranayama:

Chanting "OM":

Space for questions:

Opportunities to give feedback:

What gets in the way of you letting people in your class express their autonomy? How can you foster autonomy while still providing them with structure? What does this look like in person and online?

What does real strength as a teacher look like? How can you own your power without taking anyone else's away? How does the authority given or withheld from you in society influence this?

What are your thoughts on praxis/communal expertise? How does the idea of praxis as communal expertise tie into inclusion? What might the practice of both look like in your teaching? How might it feel to teach this way and what changes as a result?

Any additional thoughts on anything in this chapter?

Everyone Must Love Me: People Pleasing

In this section you might start to feel like I'm going the opposite direction to what I've asked you to consider thus far, and you're not wrong in that. Just as counter actions between muscle groups help create stability in the body, counter actions in our best practices help create balance in our teaching. On one hand, we see ourselves as not being better-than or above those in our classes. One the other hand, there is the need to recognize that even with this attitude, we are still a human being with personal needs who is also in a position of power. Because of this, we need some parameters to protect both ourselves and others. Boundaries have briefly come up before, here's where we get right down into them.

Repeatedly.

My Story: Everybody Loves Tori

After the ills of authority, with my shame still fresh, I decided it was time to finally "open my heart" to the people I taught. If you're not sure what that means, join the club; it's subjective expression if ever there was one. For me at the time, it made sense to swing the pendulum as far as I could in the opposite direction, towards making everything about my students. I've always inclined towards being a people pleaser in my personal life (another bullying survival strategy that stayed with me into adulthood) so I fell into it quite easily.

This was a time when I had students who really loved me. Like, loooooved me. They told me so, and I believed them (I hadn't discovered yet that being liked as a yoga teacher is actually fairly easy). There was one lady, in particular, who used to come to my classes all the time. She'd tell me on a regular basis that she thought I was the greatest gift to the world of yoga. She brought me random gifts sometimes, like pretty soap and hair products (in hindsight, maybe she just thought I needed to take better care of my hygiene). She repeatedly told me how much more love I gave to my classes compared to other teachers and how that this was helping her heal. Go me! I felt like I was on the right track (finally). After being a fake, a narcissist, and a self-righteous a-hole I was finally doing right by people. So, I kept on loving my classes with all the loving lovely love I could muster. It was an easy assumption to make—that happy people equals being a great teacher.

I made it my personal mission to make sure every person in class felt seen and left feeling better than when they'd arrived. I joked, I sang, I foot massaged, I emoted, I did everything that might work to get people to a happy zen-like place. I listened to people's life stories after class, I let people pick my brain with questions. I was as open as I could be without prying my own chest open like Hanuman. As a result of these efforts, I felt wanted by and connected to those in my classes and so I felt fulfilled by what I was doing. I was achieving all I'd ever wanted as a teacher, finally. At last, I was good at it...or I was until I became too tired to keep the love geyser going. Try as I might, I just couldn't please everyone all the time without it coming at my own expense. I didn't really realize that this is what was happening at the time—I just thought I sucked at being open due to some intrinsic character flaw. Seriously, the Dalai Lama never mentioned care fatigue in any of his books.

As an act of self-preservation, I started keeping some energy for myself rather than give it all away. After a few weeks of this, that same lady, who'd professed so many wonderful things about me, promptly told me after class one day that she wasn't coming back because I, "had no more love to give." Initially, I was devastated. I'd failed at teaching so many times…and now I was even failing at love? I was sad, and then I was really pissed off and resentful because I felt used. And eventually, as usual, the whole situation left me a bit confused; how can I be a great teacher if being a great teacher leaves me with nothing for myself?

Emotional Labour vs Teaching

I have come to believe, whole heartedly, that if you teach by showering your students with all your love and attention, you will attract very needy students and you will also likely burn out. By the way, if you're thinking this can't happen if you teach solely online, you're mistaken and you're also fortunate enough to have never had anyone slide into your DMs or inbox with their life story. How much people need you will feel really nice at first…so long as you can keep up emotionally spoon-feeding them. When you can't maintain the level of support (because we are only human) that they are accustomed to, both they and you will likely get resentful.

I confused holding space for students with doing emotional labour for them. It was an honest mistake. The difference between the two is deceivingly simple. Take teaching relaxation for example: holding space for someone to relax is acting in such a way that helps facilitate their relaxation while knowing it may/may not happen for a multitude of factors beyond our control. Doing emotional labour is taking personal responsibility for someone's ability to relax and putting the onus for the outcome chiefly on ourselves regardless of the limitations of the person or the situation. See the difference?

We all do emotional labour for ourselves—it's the work of responsibly navigating our own emotions. Taking on someone else's emotional labour means we're trying to do that work for them. It's poor emotional boundaries, that's why it's so bloody draining. The expectation that I had to make every single person in my class happy was not only unrealistic, it was self harming. The answer to my question about being a great teacher is that this is not, in fact, great teaching. It was placing the burden of people's wellbeing solely on myself. Taking on another person's inner work isn't even teaching, it's called enabling. It can feel nice but it's not healthy for anyone involved.

Your Story: How Do You Make People Love You?

Why did you initially want to be a yoga teacher? To what extent were you influenced by how you thought people would respond to you as a teacher? Does this still influence you? Why or why not? How does this influence affect your teaching?

How much is your self-worth as a teacher tied to people liking/loving you? How can this potentially lead to people pleasing behaviours and/or enabling? If you know it has, talk about the experience.

How do you respond when someone doesn't like you or your class? How do you feel emotionally and in your body?

How do you express love and compassion as a teacher? Is this sustainable for you? Is this love and compassion unconditional or with an agenda? (No. Wrong. Answer. To. This!)

Have you ever experienced emotional burn-out or care fatigue from teaching? Can you think of specific reasons why it happened? Was it preventable or not? Has anything changed as a result?

How do gender, cultural, age, skin colour, and body stereotypes affect your teaching and/or people pleasing habits and/or the people pleasing habits that others expect you to have?

What are your limits, emotional or otherwise, as a teacher? Do you tend to view these as positive or negative? Why? What has been your experience of emotional boundaries as a student and teacher of yoga?

Any other thoughts/reflections on wanting to please everyone?

Practice Emotional Boundaries

Boundaries, You'll Learn To Love 'Em

Personal boundaries are the physical, emotional, and mental guidelines established within a relationship that help everyone show up in the best possible way. They allow us to separate who we are, and what we think and feel, from the thoughts and feelings of others. As such, they are a great way protect ourselves from harmful behaviours such as manipulation, bullying, and good old enabling (thinking other's needs matter more than our own). Sounds so simple to do, right? Lordy, if I had a dollar for every time I accidentally let my boundaries slide I could drop one of my weekly classes.

One of the loveliest freedoms that comes with boundaries of the emotional variety is that we are allowed to have our feelings and other people are allowed to have theirs. No one is one hundred percent responsible for the way anyone else feels, unless, of course, their actions are the direct cause of those feelings; that's different. Bottom line, we are not responsible for the emotional well-being of the people in our classes. We can empathize, yes, but it is not our job to heal anyone's heart for them. People may occasionally convince us otherwise, especially if we have the predisposition to be a people pleaser, but we always have the choice to not go there. If we do go there out of habit, we can always choose to not go there the next time we feel pulled in that direction. Not everyone will thank you for having boundaries—I've lost students over it. No one else has outright told me I "have no love to give" (I find that story hilarious now), but there can be a feeling of me having somehow let them down as a teacher. It's tough not to take it personally, but it really does have nothing to do with us.

Emotional Boundaries While Teaching

Our role as teachers is to, as best we're able, create an environment where people are safe to express what they feel and be themselves. That's enough. And even then, there is no guarantee that they will feel safe—remember, we all have different needs and experiences. We hold space by being present with people, not by making them love us or taking responsibility for their practice. Rather than seeing each person in a class as someone to win over, we can see each person in class as someone of value. It's a teeny shift in perspective from valuing what we can potentially get from a person (we feel good because they feel good) to simply valuing that person as they are. It's an easy concept to get behind, but like anything, putting it into practice takes some skill development.

We don't simply decide one day to not use people in class to meet our emotional needs and then never do it again. The same goes for allowing other people to use us. That goes double if we are members of a marginalized group that has historically placated others as a means of survival in dominant society. The urge to follow the old patterns needs to be acknowledged, felt, and dealt with in as mature a way as we're capable of at the time. We can start by thinking about our own emotional needs as teachers and what boundaries we can put in place to meet these needs. Similar to transparency, it is us being ourselves and caring for ourselves with skill. We then get to practice putting those boundaries in place and, in doing so, get a better sense of if they are, in fact, what we need. Boundaries aren't set in stone, they are allowed to shift and change as we shift and change. As nice as it would be to instantly and undeniably know exactly what boundaries we need and when, life just doesn't work that way.

I've already told you about my realizations around being touched and adjusted while practicing. I uphold this necessary boundary while teaching in several ways: while I'm usually all about hugs, I do not hug students on days when I do not feel like being touched, and I mostly teach through demonstration and verbal cues rather than hands-on adjustments. It's true that this approach does not work for all people, and that's fine. I'm as accommodating as I can be in my teaching style without compromising my own well-being (not the same as never challenging my comfort zones or personal beliefs).

It's worth giving people the benefit of the doubt when it comes to implementing new boundaries in your teaching. When I first started implementing my "no hugs if I don't want hugs", rule I was concerned how some people would take it. One person I know who absolutely loved hugs after class was the first to test my new boundary. It wasn't even an issue. All I had to say was that I wasn't in a mood for hugging and that was that—we started fist bumping on those days instead. It doesn't always play out like that, but sometimes it does.

Another example: I like talking with people before class but, like clockwork, I always excuse myself to the washroom or off-screen for five minutes before class starts. I don't really do much while I'm away from the class—I focus on my breath, look into my own eyes in the mirror, or do whatever else feels right as a way to ground myself in those few minutes. Taking this time before every class is a simple way of showing up for myself that helps me not get swept away by old patterns while teaching.

Being grounded is always helpful as a teacher, but it's a life-saver on those odd occasions when a new person shows up and looks at me halfway through class like I'm the worst teacher on the planet because I don't teach how they like to practice. Those folks inevitably happen. There's not much to be done apart from not taking their preferences personally. A big aspect of emotional boundaries is not allowing other people's reactions to us define who we are. This includes setting personal boundaries to protect yourself from social power imbalances and biases that trickle into the classroom. We have a responsibility for our students but we don't owe them anything that does us harm.

Personal boundaries help us feel safe and when we feel safe we are better equipped to leave our comfort zone and grow. It's more complex than the old self-help metaphor, "you have to put on your own oxygen mask before you help anyone else with theirs." It's more like an EMT or first responder situation—you have to make your own well-being a priority, not because you're more important than the person you are helping, but because you both are going to be worse off if you don't look after yourself. Teaching is a balance of simultaneously owning what we need in order to do our job while not making those needs the sole focus of the class. The people in our class have needs of their own that are just as valid as ours. Sound conflicting? It can be. Personally, I now have a whole list of other teachers to recommend to people if what I'm offering isn't what they're looking for. People's needs and our boundaries won't always mix. When they don't, it's nothing personal; there are a thousand other yoga teachers a person can go to if they want a hug each and every class.

Your Practice: How Will You Bring Emotional Boundaries Into Your Teaching

How does showing up for people as they are, without an emotional agenda or making them a means to an end feel in your body? How does it change your interactions with others and the amount of energy they require? How does this differ from trying to please people? Describe how you feel/know the difference and how you can be aware if it in the future.

What emotional boundaries would serve you as a teacher in the following areas? What are ways you can start to put these boundaries into practice while teaching? Start by brainstorming and then reread to see what feels true for you. It's cool if you change your mind on how to do this after you try it out (you likely will and that's a good thing).

Before and after class:

While teaching online and in-person:

Social media and messaging:

With people who want to monopolize your energy and attention:

With people who put you on a pedestal:

With people who do not like the way you teach:

Outside of the classroom (personal life):

As a student:

Other areas that are important to you:

Based on your answers to the earlier question about how gender, cultural, age, skin colour and body stereotypes/biases affect your experience of teaching, what specific boundaries can you put in place to protect yourself from harmful stereotypes/biases causing you harm as a teacher?

What does healthy expression of love look like in your class? Explain the difference between emotional labour and holding space in you own words.

A Little Too Open: Yoga Crushes and Teacher/Student Relationships

Before we go into this one, a heads up that we are going to wade into the murky waters of professional boundaries as they pertain to sex. I want to clarify that this is not about shaming sexual empowerment or preference, it's about the misuse of sexuality. I also want to say that if you have ever been sexually harassed or abused by a teacher or student a) that person was completely in the wrong, b) feel free to skip this section because we gain nothing by forcing ourselves through triggering content, and c) that person really was completely, utterly, and absolutely in the wrong.

My Story: I May Be Kinda Sorta Available

The first regular studio class I ever taught, almost a year to the day after my wannabe fake guru debacle, was a Fridays at 5:30pm time slot. It was a notoriously hard class to fill and it wasn't going well. I was still new to teaching and was very insecure about what I was doing (yoga teacher armour fully in use). I resolved that if getting people to come to the class for the yoga wasn't gonna happen, I was gonna have to do something else to get them through the door. At the time I called it being "really friendly". In retrospect, it was too friendly.

What are the boundaries of the teacher/student relationship? Where's the line between being personable and being unprofessional? Can you form personal relationships with the people you teach outside of the classroom? Opinions vary, a lot. It's inevitable and great that people we have a lot in common with end up coming to our classes, and so friendly relationships naturally develop. The question is, where do we draw the line as to what sort of relationship we can or can't have with people who we also teach?

My curt opinion on all this is, "teaching ain't tinder." The long version is a bit more complicated.

For starters, we have good old fashioned yoga crushes. They happen all the time and, more often than not, they are harmless. There's nothing wrong with crushing on a teacher, be it romantic or otherwise. They're this great person who teaches you cool stuff and helps you feel good—how could you not crush on them? The danger comes when we, as the teacher, don't have the resources to skillfully handle the situation. Let's face it, how to maturely handle someone crushing on you or vice versa is not always likely to be included in a 200 hour YTT. We're mostly left to use our own best judgement, and nothing clouds judgement like sexual attraction.

Now, I have never crossed the romantic line with someone I have taught. The "No Hanky Panky" rule of my social work days was so imbedded in my consciousness that I just couldn't. That said, I have definitely wanted to. I have also most definitely put "the vibe" out there. And I have most definitely exploited people's attraction to me in order to fill a room and feel good about myself. I own all of it.

Back to my very, very, very friendly class. It started being predominantly filled by divorced men in their early forties. It wasn't my intention to be that specific but I guess the flirty vibe I was putting out there just happened to appeal to a very certain type. A type who showed up eagerly every Friday to hang on my every word and talk about Pink Floyd albums.

For most of my life up to that point, I'd been romantically awkward and insecure, so to have a room full of people looking at me like I was a yogic goddess was intoxicating, even if I had no romantic inclination towards most of them. I didn't see anything wrong with it, at first. The attention made me feel wanted and appreciated, and, in turn, I felt like a more confident yoga teacher. I know, again with the misguided confidence thing.

After about four months it started feeling weird. They weren't coming for my yoga teaching, they were coming because I was flirting with them and giving them questionable attention. It was not really about yoga for anyone involved—we were just a bunch of folks wanting attention from each other. By using what God gave me to fill a room I was basically saying to myself that I wasn't good enough to fill a room without it. It's a common trap for any teacher but especially those of us with a very feminine identify; we are conditioned to think we need to have, and rely on, sexual appeal and charm to do well, and in doing so, easily lose sight of our capabilities. I stopped doing it. Personally, it was akin to turning off a light switch in my brain but for some it can take a commendable amount self-restraint to change this pattern. As expected, most of the guys left. In time, as I grew into a better teacher, other people came to take their place who were more interested in yoga and platonic community.

I can't speak to the intentions of anyone who has come to a class since, but I know that on my end there are no mixed signals. I can teach in-person or online in a pair of hotpants and sports bra and know exactly what I am and am not putting out there. That's not to say that signals can't still get misread, but I know where I stand and have learned how to handle the attention if it arises.

We Are Not Who People See

The error is not in the attraction (crushes happen, and from both sides). The error is in thinking that these crushes are based in reality. I'm sorry, but we yoga teachers are just not that special. People in our classes may think we are the best and love us, sure, but it's up to us as teachers to keep our feet on the ground and not get swept away by it. Who we are in the role of teacher is not the entirety who we are— what people perceive in class is not the whole picture. Yes, we try to be transparent and all that, but I can't come in bitching about my landlord, the weird rash on my back, or my visa bill. Those in my classes get the parts of me that best serve the situation, but not the whole. People are crushing on a mix of the aspects of my personality I most embody when I'm teaching and the image they project onto me based on their subjective experience. That goes double for online classes and social media. I remember being absolutely head over heels about a yoga teacher I had while in university; when I got to know him years later as a fellow teacher, he wasn't at all the person/personal saviour I'd made him out to be (I actually didn't like him all that much).

In social work and clinical settings, we call the unconscious act of the client projecting their wants and needs onto the therapist transference. A simplified example would be a person in therapy beginning to see their therapist as a parental figure and reacting to them as they would a parent. Transference can occur just as easily in yoga as it can in therapy. In this case, it's a student thinking that their yoga teacher is their ideal romantic partner because every time they interact with this teacher, they feel great (likely, because they are doing yoga). It's not real, but it's easy for people to believe it is. If, as a teacher, we employ a lot of charm, fake persona, narcissism, and/or emotional labour while we teach, the reality is going to be even more skewed and the basis for romantic attachment even more false.

Power Imbalance is Not Sexy

But it feels great, doesn't it? It's easy to look down on this sort of behaviour until someone is looking at us like we're God's gift to humankind. Just like sexual attraction, positions of power have a sneaky way of clouding our judgement. In that instance, especially if the attraction is mutual, it's easy to convince ourselves we are the exception to the "No Hanky Panky" rule.

There are exceptions, of course, but those exceptions have something that most do not: both participants on equal ground. What does that mean? Well, imagine someone comes to your class once and then you run into them on the street a month later. You strike up a casual conversation that you both contribute to (no one is teaching anyone anything), both feel a wee spark and decide to go for coffee sometime. There's no teacher/student or uneven power dynamic— that's equal ground. Now imagine someone who has been diligently practicing with you for the last year and who you know (or think you know) has a bit of a crush on "teacher you". You decide you are interested in perusing them and so start flirting with them and eventually ask them out after one of your classes. What are differences between the first situation and this one? I'm not looking for a right answer, just that your wheels start turning on this.

Many people come to yoga searching for something. It's easy to fall into the trap of thinking that "special something" resides in an external source or person rather than within themselves. Sometimes this takes the shape of teacher worship. Other times, or often simultaneously, it can take the shape of romantic attraction. This is why, in my opinion, teacher-student sexual relationships are 99.9% of the time a terrible, awful, don't-go-there idea. To hold space for someone while they are vulnerable in class and then later use that same connection as a gateway to romance or sex is a misuse of power and a breach of any trust previously built in the relationship. It is part of our responsibility as the teacher to draw that line and keep it, as difficult as it might be. The bond of a teacher and a student is a precious thing. It deserves our care and respect.

No matter what, the moment we find ourselves at the front of a yoga class we are in a position of influence and power. That's just the way it is. While this power imbalance can be lessened, it will always be there and it will always affect how everyone else in the room relates to us. Awareness of this and its potential consequences for everyone involved is how we handle these situations with skill. Another way to say all of that is, *when you are in a position of power you have a duty to not act like a creep.*

Your Story: Ever Crossed a Line?

I've been fairly gender-neutral in this section for the sake of scope and brevity. I acknowledge that this limits some VERY important aspects of this discussion. Please get as gender specific as you need to in your reflections—especially if your experience of gender makes your story completely different from mine. If you feel like you don't need to bring up gender at all, that's also worth reflecting on.

Where is the line for you between being personable and being unprofessional? Why and what is this based on?

Do you form friendships with students that extend outside of yoga? How do you decide when this is a good idea or a bad idea? Does how you act in these friendships differ from other relationships?

Have you ever slept with or dated a person you also taught? What was your motivation? What was the outcome for you both (in any/all instances)? If you don't know what the outcome was for them, why don't you know?

Have you or do you use sexuality or flirting to fill classes? Do you see it as problematic or not? What potential repercussions are there for you and/or others? What does the difference between sexual empowerment and misuse of sexuality look and feel like for you? Can you articulate it in a way that helps guide your actions as a teacher?

Have you ever been hit-on or sexualized by someone in a position of power? How did you respond and how did that differ from what you actually felt in that moment? What do you think about that situation now? What lessons can you take from that experience and apply to your teaching?

What other stories, thoughts and/or reflections do you have on this topic based on your own unique life experience?

Where do you think your line is in teacher/students relationships? Can you think of times you've upheld this line and other times when you have not? Has your opinion on this topic changed over time? What it means to you to be on "equal ground" with someone?

Practice Professional Relationship Boundaries and Work/Life Balance

Yay! More Boundaries

The key to having solid boundaries of any kind is a sense of identity and self-worth. Like all people, we teachers have our insecurities—maybe even more-so being that many of us are overly introspective and somewhat introverted. It's my very subjective theory that, for many of us, our role as a teacher is a way to interact with others that feels safer and more in control than our normal, everyday selves. We're more confident when people see us as a teacher because there is that little step up from them to us. We also know they assume the best about us. Add to this the fact that teaching can take a lot of time and effort that comes at the expense of a separate social life, and hitting on folks at the yoga studio is a little more understandable. Understandable, but still not cool.

Sexual Boundaries

As illustrated earlier, when we seek to engage in romantic behaviour with people we teach, we are doing so from a place of authority. Being the killjoy that I am, it's my stance that the very reasons we feel more confident to act in this manner are the exact same reasons we shouldn't do it. We feel elevated and in charge...but what then does that say about the other person in this situation? Likely, they feel less powerful. In some cases, that disempowerment might even be the primary basis for their attraction. This dynamic can be especially true if you're a male and/or masculine teacher relating to a female/femme student as it mirrors gender power imbalances found on a societal level.

My favourite definition of professional boundaries is that they create space between one person's power and another's vulnerability. Setting professional boundaries around teacher/student sexual relationships protects us from abusing our power despite our best intentions. To know where our line needs to be takes all we've learned about ourselves in the previous sections and over the span of our lives—we need to know our potential pitfalls if we are going to create a model for teaching that doesn't feed into them. For example: if we know we easily fall into overusing charm and sometimes struggle with upholding emotional boundaries (that's me!), it's probably a great idea to have a very hard line (no flirting or dating, and friendships made with a whole lotta discernment) we know never to cross.

And Another Thing About Boundaries

Sometimes the sexual boundary dynamic is the total opposite—a person in class is really attracted to you and continually does not respect the boundaries you are trying to set. My first experience with this was with a man who organized a corporate class for me. He was new to yoga and socially awkward; a yoga crush blossomed. I was at a point where I could recognize this and not feed into it, but my usual approach was not enough to get the message across. I shied away from addressing the matter head-on because I hoped he'd just get over it. He didn't. He began withholding my paycheque until I came to see him personally to get it. When I picked it up, he would remind me how his mother, who also worked there, was in charge of me getting paid or not paid. After a couple months it was clear that he was not going to back off on his own, he was going to keep escalating. The situation got unsettling when he got my home address and phone number off my invoice and started texting me whenever he just happened to be in my area. With emotional support from a friend, I resolved to sit him down and draw a very solid line: I don't date students and if you cannot accept that and change your behaviour then you can no longer organize or attend my classes. If he didn't listen, I resolved to tell on him to his mom. To his credit, he heard me. With, I might add, apparent horror that our romance had existed entirely in his head. He gave up organizing the class and never attended it again.

Professional boundaries create space between one person's power and another's vulnerability, including when the person who is vulnerable is us. And if that boundary is too big to hold alone, we can always ask for support. Believing we have to always do it all on our own is just self-imposed dogma.

Boundaries for Teacher/Student Friendships

I do take less of a hard line with friendships. Whatever side of the friendship we are on, it still benefits us to keep an eye on transference and power imbalance leftover from the classroom that may leak into the friendship. Notice behaviours such as always giving your former (or current) student advice, if scheduling hang-outs always revolves around your schedule and not theirs, does the social influence go both ways (healthy) or are you doing all the influencing (unhealthy)? These are just some signs of a potential power imbalance. Any of these being present doesn't mean you need to end the friendship, just check yourself, talk to your friend, and take action to do better. If you're in the opposite role in this situation, ask yourself if the friendship is beneficial to you. If it is and you want to continue it, do some googling around emotional boundaries in friendships and then have a talk with your friend about it.

As an aside, if this whole student/teacher relationship situation happens in the reverse order; partners, friends, family members coming to our classes, we need to be aware of a whole different strain of boundaries and assumptions. The familiarity we have with these people can easily lead to us taking liberties with them that might not be what they need or want while they practice. A friend may love joking around with us off the mat but while on it they may prefer we don't draw the class's attention to them while they practice. We may feel very comfortable adjusting a family member but that does not mean that they feel like being touched that particular day. It's best never to assume based on interactions outside of the classroom, just ask.

Create A Life Off The Mat

One of the best ways we can help ourselves keep our interpersonal and sexual boundaries is by not looking to get all our social needs met through teaching. Being a yoga teacher is often very solitary work. It's easy to run around expending all our social energy on our classes and leave very little for our personal life. In this situation, it's tempting to let our loneliness get the best of us. I honestly think loneliness is where a lot of boundary crossing comes from.

We are social creatures and, while social interaction is necessary for developing that sense ofdentity and worth that are key to having boundaries, these needs cannot be met by solely by the people in our classes. Remember the previous section; the people in our classes are not a means to an end; emotional, sexual, or otherwise. We need to leave room for a meaningful social life outside of the classroom. As much as I have tried to not be overly prescriptive in this book, I will say that a healthy social life is a necessity for everyone—however that looks for them. Walking into a class with our social needs already met (as best we can on any given day) makes it easier to simply teach. One effective way to save the energy needed to have said social life is by applying the emotional boundaries we learned about in the previous section. I like to think of it as always holding a bit of energy back in classes so I can keep it for myself.

Your Practice: How Will You Bring Relationship Boundaries Into Your Teaching?

Based on your history, personality, life experience, and what you've learned about yourself in the previous sections, what boundaries do you want/need to have with the people you teach?

What's the line you won't cross with someone in your class? Why? What steps can you take to keep these boundaries?

Write your boundaries for each of the following areas as they relate to teacher/student relationships:

Friendship:

Sex life:

Romance/dating:

Social outings/engagement:

What other interpersonal and sexual boundaries do you want/need to set based on socialized power dynamics and where these dynamics try to place you in society?

How can you create space to ensure your needs are met, without relying on your students, in the following areas:

Friendship:

Sex life:

Romance/dating:

Social outings/engagement:

Saviourism: Unqualified Advice and Fixing People

My Story: Just Call Me Jesus

Oh, saviourism.

The sweet nectar of knowing what's best for everyone. Is there anything more deeply satisfying?

That glorious feeling of knowing exactly what another person needs and being able to articulate it to them in such a way that denotes just how much we know about their situation. It's a bit of a high, ain't it? It can make us feel like the greatest teacher in the whole damn world regardless of whether our advice actually benefits anyone.

I often joked when I was a social worker that," Solving other people's problems is a great way of avoiding your own." It was funny because it was, in my case, true. One of the primary reasons I quit being a social worker, other than my inability to sit at a desk eight hours a day, was the realization that I liked the saviour-like image of being a social worker more than I liked the actual work itself. And, if it wasn't the case already, this was bound to eventually make me terrible, and dangerous to others, at my job. Here's why: being primarily motivated by my own self image meant that my working relationships with clients were inevitably going to be about feeding my own ego rather than the efficacy of what I was doing. Obviously, this was not the point of being a social worker. I'd say the same is true for being a yoga teacher.

I thought I left my saviour habit behind me when I quit social work, but a month later there I was in Rishikesh trying to save everybody and their monkey with healing sounds I couldn't pronounce. This started an embarrassingly long era in my early years of teaching where I loved sounding like a therapist but refused to admit I needed therapy. I was giving advice based on personal experience, a handful of yoga trainings and meditation retreats, and a social work degree that should have taught me enough to know I was not qualified to be a therapist (something I conveniently forgot when no longer around other social workers). I'm less embarrassed by this now since discovering that giving unqualified and/or unsolicited advice is not altogether uncommon among yoga teachers.

I would read a book by the latest and greatest self-help author and teach their ideas in class as if they were the new universal gospel. Someone in class would be having a tough day and I'd spout out a solution based on Ayurveda, in which I had a solid thirty hours of training, without knowing anything about that particular person or their situation. And, I saved the best for last, I got interested in yoga for trauma and started teaching practices I'd seen online as if I'd been properly trained in them. That last one sounds particularly bad, and it is. It also happens all the time. Now, learning new things to teach from social media, blogs (do people still blog?), and through other classes is as common as the smell of luon fabric in a yoga studio change room, and that's fine. We all do it. However, how do we decide what is and isn't fair game?

Yoga for trauma seemed like a very straightforward concept...until I took the time to really learn the concept. Yes, I had lots of teaching experience, and yes, I was most certainly capable of teaching yoga for trauma, but neither of these meant that I was qualified to teach this without actual training and/or study. That people liked what I was teaching was also not a reliable gauge of its quality or safety because they all assumed I knew what I was doing. People enjoying what we teach is great but it's similar to people liking their yoga teacher—it's not always an accurate indicator of actual benefit.

The fact that I had trauma of my own was not in and of itself a qualification. I knew at this point that I had trauma but figured that years of yoga combined with my professional background meant it was more or less taken care of. Sadly, without the professional help I needed to begin healing my own nervous system, my attempts to heal others were causing me harm and re-traumatizing me. A fact that I would have known if I'd taken the time to train and dig deeper into what yoga for trauma actually was. Remember my social work joke? Well the yoga for trauma version goes like this, "Attempting to heal other people's trauma is a great way to avoid healing your own."

I WILL Fix You

Think back on the teachers you've known who were always giving you advice; how much of their assistance was actually about you and how much was about them? Personally, in retrospect I see distinct differences between the advice given for the sake of advice (seldom helped me and often made things worse) and receiving guidance from my teachers. The same is true when I look back at my own behaviour.

Saviourism in this way is wanting to help people more for our own satisfaction with ourselves than for their benefit. Like many of our previous "How Nots", it stems from the normal human inclination to want to feel good about ourselves and what we do, but we go about it in an embellished and potentially harmful way. Our desire to be taken seriously and impact people's lives can lead us to do and say things that, in the long run, have the opposite effect. It's ridiculously easy to present a basic understanding and/or personal opinion dressed up like a teaching and not even realize it. Not that there's anything wrong with basic knowledge and opinions, we just save everyone a lot of trouble when we call them what they are.

It can be a bit like codependency and enabling behaviours; it is about wanting to be needed. The difference is in the narratives. Codependency usually believes that we have to give people whatever they want so they'll need us, saviourism believes that what people need is whatever we want for them.

Sometimes We Just Get Excited

I think a lot of unqualified teaching/advice has to do with us simply getting excited about something new we've learned and rushing to teach it before we are ready. This happened to me a couple years ago when I decided to teach a class based on a Ted Talk I saw about mirror neurons. Mirror neurons are a neuron that fires when we both do an action ourselves and see an action performed by another and so, potentially, create collective learning. It's that whole interconnectedness of all life thing and it got me really excited. So excited that I brought it up while I was chatting with a professor of Early Childhood Development before a class I'd decided to teach entirely on mirror neurons. She was really nice about cutting it apart. Apparently mirror neurons have been proven to exist in animals but there is no way to prove exactly what they do or if they exist in humans. The possibility of them is fascinating and exciting, but it is still only a theory being explored. Don't worry if you're a fan—they likely do exist in some capacity, there's simply still a lot of unknowns. She went on to explain how the Ted Talk phenomena, while great, is best viewed as an exciting intro to new ideas, not as hard research. Sometimes researchers also get excited about new possibilities and make claims that might not be proven fact. Point taken. Always look for multiple sources and different opinions. I still taught a class on collective learning, I just centred it around the importance of learning from each other, the value of which I had just experienced 10 minutes prior.

Big Hands vs Little Hands

I see two ways to be a yoga teacher; a big hands teacher and a little hands teacher. No, I don't mean in terms of adjustments, that's creepy. Big hands carry people. We scoop them up with all the attention, know-how, and advice we can muster in the hopes that they'll love us dearly for it. But is that what it means to be a good yoga teacher? Are we really helping anyone when we spoon feed them our answers (right or wrong)?

I did a private class with a yoga teacher in Varanasi who was a big hands teacher. It was his view that each posture had to be held for one minute for it to be beneficial—even if I wasn't holding it on my own. It was an odd lesson; this studio was literally a padded room, so balancing was extremely difficult. I remember him holding me up in dancers pose telling me that I didn't need to do anything because being in the shape was the benefit. Now, Kriya Yoga is not my specialty so I can't say much at all about the intent or the outcome of the class. I share the story not to start a debate between styles of yoga, but as an illustration of what I mean by big hands teaching.

In most, not all, class situations, it is a bit pointless for a teacher to do more work than a student in order for the student to hold a balance posture. Sure, we can offer support but what is point of us doing dancers pose for them? From a biomechanical point of view there really isn't any. Even if you are a fan of very hands-on adjustments, I think you'd agree with me that the intention is eventually the person being adjusted will need you less and less. The benefit of the person doing the activity is in the experience of attempting to do it— wobbling, falling, frustration, etc—not the end position itself. If we take that experience away in order to get them to where we think they should be, they miss out on the benefits of getting there themselves. Another example: we can tell someone that they need to drop their front ribs and help put them into that position to show them what we mean, but this is not the same as them experiencing what it feels like to drop their front ribs using their own body awareness and skill. The point of teaching then, is to help them find this experience for themselves and learn to apply it in a way that works for them.

The same is true for the intellectual, emotional, and spiritual aspects in a class. We support, but we don't need to do the work for them or tell them where it should lead. Remember way back when I said we learn to bypass from our teachers? This right here is how you break that cycle. One of the best ways to discourage spiritual bypassing is to start resisting the urge to tell people where their road should lead. Maybe doing yoga will change someone's personal habits, but I don't know which ones. Maybe doing yoga will change their relationships, but what that will look like for someone is beyond me. Maybe they'll get up into a handstand some day, but maybe it doesn't even matter.

Now the alternative, what I call small hands teaching. Small hands teaching is the 100% hand-over-heart belief that people are resilient, capable, and their own best teachers via their own praxis—with or without us. It's taking our practices of empathy and autonomy and amping them up with a little something called unconditional positive regard. Simply put, this is a choice to always focus on the capability and competence of those we teach. Especially when they don't see it themselves. Small hands are there to monitor, support, and facilitate growth. It's a gentle touch here and there to help guide someone as they move, grow, and change in the way that works for them—no pulling, no prodding, and no carrying. Their practice is their own, not ours. This is a view that is impossible to hold if we still buy into pedestals, narcissism, or being an absolute authority figure.

I can't speak for anyone else on this, but personally, the more I attended to my own healing, the less I wanted to try healing everyone else. I don't believe in anyone ever being "completely healed"; in my experience that is just wishful thinking and bypassing. I do, however, fully and absolutely endorse continually working on our stuff—for our own sake and for that of our students.

Your Story: Saved Anyone Lately?

How do you want to be seen/ regarded as a teacher? Is this image key to you continuing to teach? To what extent does it motivate your decisions and choices? What are the pros and cons of this self-image?

Have you ever been given advice by a teacher that you later found out was unqualified or misrepresented? Have you even been given advice that was harmful to you? Is this a habit that you've taken into your own teaching?

Do you give advice to people you teach? What is your motivation for giving advice and what are the outcomes (if any)? Have you ever given life advice based on personal experience/preference to a student? What was your motivation for doing so? What was the outcome?

Have you ever taught something based on excitement rather than knowledge? What are your thoughts on teaching subjects you are only just learning about yourself? How can you tell the difference between self-doubt and knowing your own limits in this situation?

Are there particular topics you like to give advice on more than others? Is this because you are more knowledgeable in these areas? Is it because you are more opinionated? Or is there another motivation?

What is your experience, if any, with big vs small hands teaching? What was the effect on you as a student and a teacher?

How do you determine the needs of people who come to your classes, if at all? How subjective is this judgement call? Have you found way to make it more objective, if possible?

Think back to your own teachers. Who was the most effective at helping you discover your own practice and who was the least effective. Why? What skills and qualities did they utilize that you want to mimic?

What has been your experience with "solving other people's problems is a great way of avoiding your own," as a teacher and as a student? Remember, hindsight is 20/20 so don't be too hard on yourself.

Practice Knowing Your Scope
and Staying in Your Lane

Scope of Practice

Scope of practice is a tool for defining the areas in which we are qualified to function professionally (in this case teach). If your heart just jumped into your throat because you think you don't have any, I assure that this is not the case; that reaction is likely just some good old imposter syndrome that we will get to later. Staying in our lane is similar to staying within our scope. The term is usually used as a recommendation against sharing thoughts and/or opinions on a subject about which we have insufficient knowledge or understanding. For example, I'm stepping out of my lane/scope if I position myself as any kind of expert on the impact of cultural appropriation on Indigenous people because I have absolutely no experience of being a person who is Indigenous. Hence, the referrals in that section to qualified Indigenous teachers.

We're going to define our own scope right now with an exercise that breaks down our knowledge onto four categories:

Areas I have a lot of experiential and/or trained knowledge of:

Areas I have a little knowledge/training in but am interested in:

Areas I know little to nothing about:

Areas I have a lot of opinions about:

Here's some of mine as an example:

Areas I have a lot of experiential and/or trained knowledge of:

Personally, I have a lot of experiential and trained knowledge of:
trauma informed yoga (yes, I know what I'm doing now), anatomy,
biomechanics, Advaita Vedanta philosophy and mediation, and a
mash-up of different asana styles, social work related fields like
interpersonal dynamics, best practices, mental health, group
facilitation, addictions, social and political structures, social justice
issues (as an ally, not through personal experience).

Areas I have a little knowledge/training in but am interested in:

I have little knowledge/training but an interest in mirror neurons
(hahaha), acupressure, dietary requirements, energy healing, cult
dynamics, therapeutic interventions, prenatal specific yoga, Yogic and
Buddhist philosophies that I do not personally practice and the
Eastern cultures where these practices originated, marketing
strategies, yoga for specific disabilities and physical conditions, and
yoga therapy.

Areas I know nothing about:

I know very little/nothing about injury assessment/diagnosis,
acupuncture, massage, physical and mental illness
diagnosis/treatment, self-help and life coaching protocols,
chiropractic adjustments, Kriya Yoga along with a whole list of yoga
styles/lineages I've never practiced, Indigenous spiritual practices
apart from yoga, aromatherapy, physiotherapy protocols, and first-
hand experience of systemic discrimination or oppression. (This list
could go on forever so I'm sticking to what is most relevant to
teaching yoga)

Areas I have a lot of opinions about:

I have a lot of opinions about (this can include topics from the other
categories) energetic healing, politics, self-care, the commodification
of yoga/health, marketing strategies, Kundalini Yoga, Yogic and

Buddhist philosophy, the New Thought Movement and manifestation theory, healthy vs unhealthy lifestyle choices, traditional asana, and how to teach yoga (insert winky face emoji).

Your Practice, Part One: Find Your Scope

Now you:

Areas I have a lot of experiential and/or trained knowledge of:

Areas I have a little knowledge/training in but am interested in:

Areas I know little to nothing about:

Areas I have a lot of opinions about (can include topics from other lists):

We know a lot. We also don't know a lot. We also have a lot of opinions. It's all fine. The trick is knowing which is which and what we have the qualifications and experience to teach. I mention experiential knowledge again because I don't believe we always need to complete a training in order to teach something; someone who has been meditating for two decades but has no formal training will likely have far more knowledge than a 30 hour meditation training graduate.

The trick of knowing our scope, and staying in our lane, is simply owning what we do know and owning what we don't; "I don't know," is a perfectly reasonable response to any question while teaching. So is, "I don't know but that is interesting and I'm going to look into it," and so is, "I don't know, does anyone else here have any ideas?" You'd be amazed how smart people in classes are when given a chance to shine.

Opinions are nothing to shy away from. Often it is our opinions that make us interesting to people. Without our unique personality and thoughts we are right back up to section one with pretending to be what we think a yoga teacher should be. Have your opinions but own them as your own subjective opinions, not fact. For example: I'm not all that keen on eating an Ayurvedic diet. Eating for my dosha never worked all that well for me in practice and also tended to feed the part of my brain that likes to micromanage my eating habits. This is a subjective opinion, based solely on my own experience and preferred practice; it doesn't apply to anyone but me. If someone in class asks me about doshas I can tell them the basics and share that it's not my cup of tea while also encouraging them to read up on it themselves and make up their own mind about it. We do not all need to have the same opinions to get along (sameness and unity are not the same). In this way, being ourselves can lend itself to encouraging others to do the same.

Restraint Is a Virtue

So, there's knowing your scope, that's one part. The second is resolving to not go outside of it— this is usually the harder part. It can be really hard to keep our mouths shut when we think we know what's best for people. Especially if we are slightly knowledgeable in the area of concern. It's even harder when we know that they're interested in, and will likely believe, our opinion-tainted advice. This might not be such an issue if it's two friends sitting on a couch but when it's a yoga teacher giving out mental health or dietary advice it can be a disaster.

As you read the remainder of this section I want you to keep in mind the list of things you know a lot about and the list of things you are very opinionated about. Get extra curious about how you behave on topics that fall into both lists.

Like personal boundaries, professional boundaries help us to feel safe in a healthy way. Setting parameters for ourselves isn't sexy or all that fun, but practicing accountability is one of the ways we learn how to trust ourselves as teachers. How can we ever hope to gain real confidence in our abilities, without relying on authority and manipulation, if deep down we know we are talking out of our ass half of the time? There is no better cure for imposter syndrome than giving yourself permission to not know everything and be everything to everyone. This is how we as teachers also benefit from small hands teaching that supports people instead of carrying them. This approach may not always be welcome, some people really like being carried, but is the cost to them and us worth it? As teachers, we are not *insert name of preferred deity*. And we don't have to be, thank *insert name of preferred deity*.

Real empowerment as a teacher requires us to take a step back from our want to control and our desire to be needed by students.

A Beautiful Alternative

Even if the advice we are giving is right on the mark, consider this: when it comes to self-growth how many of us have had deep insights arise from being told by another person what that deep insight should be? Chances are not many of us. Personally, I have been told things about myself that were true, but these truths didn't mean anything until I was in a place where I was able to realize them for myself. What helped me get to that place was not the teachers who told me where I needed to go but the teachers who accepted me where I was, as I was.

There is immense power in being able to take interest in whoever is in front of us without needing to change them. I'm not talking about staring at anyone's aura or into their deeper self, I mean being with them, as they are, without any need for embellishment or romanticization. Think back on your own experiences as a student; what helped you more when you were in need of support, a person who immediately told you what you should do or the person who unflinchingly sat with you and let you be exactly how you were in that moment? Seeing people and being present with them is often all that is required for us to have the positive impact on others we so deeply desire. Presence is the ground in which healthy relationships grow. It's just so ordinary that the profoundness of it as a practiced skill easily gets forgotten amid flashier yoga talents. Combined with unconditional positive regard and guidance that strengthens people in coming to their own insights; being present with people is one of the greatest gifts we can offer as a yoga teacher.

This change in perspective can be a tricky shift to navigate, but in the end, again, it's less work and, I believe, ultimately more fulfilling. An example: I teach a lot of people with back pain due to chronic conditions. There's a lot of info out there on back pain, I've read a lot of this information, however I'm still qualified to diagnose almost nothing when it comes to back pain (scope of practice). When someone approaches me in pain, my instant reaction is to think back on everything I do know and find something (anything!) I can offer to make it go away (big hands). That impulse isn't wrong, but it places all my attention on me fixing the condition and not on the person. So instead, I take a step back and listen to them (small hands). And I listen to them without any agenda. It's an easy, common slide in any helping profession to listen to someone only so they'll do what we say later—that's manipulation. We can all do better than that.

Having no agenda opens us up to a whole spectrum of possibilities that don't exist if we decide we know what someone needs. Sometimes I have insight to offer on someone's back pain, but I wait and I ask questions before I suggest anything. Maybe they've already tried everything I would recommend. Maybe I have no idea what their back needs but I can support them in other ways. Maybe we put our heads together and come up something new to try. Maybe they know exactly what they need and are attempting to tell me what that is. Maybe all they really wanted was someone to hear what they had to say.

Your Practice, Part Two: How Will You
Both Own Your Lane and Stay In It?

What skills and talents do you have to offer people as a teacher? Intellectually, experientially, emotionally? How do these talents come together to form your unique teaching style? What are your responsibilities to yourself and students as you offer these gifts?

What's NOT your responsibility as a yoga teacher? How does it feel to name and own what's not your responsibility?

How would you describe your scope as a yoga teacher in your own words? How would you describe staying in your lane as a yoga teacher? How does it feel to know and own this? Can it be a source of empowerment rather than self-judgement?

Go back to your expertise and opinions lists. How can you create professional boundaries that separate them enough that people are not likely to confuse one with the other? If it's an overlap item, how do you separate your opinion from your knowledge?

How can staying in your lane while guiding and supporting students help you to not act on harmful stereotypes, biases, and societal-based beliefs? Respond to any of the following that do not affect you personally. Hint: this might mean NOT doing certain things.

Racism:

Fatphobia:

Ableism (including mental illness and eating disorders):

Homophobia and Transphobia:

Classism:

Sexism:

How can you balance excitement with restraint?

What is it like, in person or online, to see and hear the people you are teaching? Online is different for sure, but it's possible. Perhaps think about how you might see/hear people in light of current events that affect us all.

How will you commit to your healing/self-work? Focus on tangible and realistic ways to support yourself, we don't need to fix ourselves either, right? What role can community play in this?

It's All Crap: Disillusionment and Existential Burnout

My Story: Turns Out It Was All Bullshit

It's hard to acknowledge the limitations and errors of our modern yoga world without getting cynical about it. I know a lot of people who have quit teaching temporarily and permanently when they got to this stage of the game. Others, understandably, jump ship and move on to something else to meet their movement and/or spiritual needs. And then there are those of us who get stuck there because we don't know where else to go. We get hard on yoga, hard on others, and hard on ourselves.

Disillusionment hit me hard in 2015. My malcontent started with not being able to bend over for two years because my hamstrings were so wrecked and ended with realizing just how much of my meagre teaching income had gone towards health cleanses that hadn't done a damn thing. I had tried each and every misinformed method I could find for being a "good" yogi and yet I continued to feel like a disgruntled failure. I'd paid through the nose for training after training as sensibilities and trends continuously shifted and none had brought me the lucidity they promised. I was broke, I was tired, and I was burnt-out. It was a chore to not roll my eyes at anything related to yoga.

I think my crowning moment as a disillusioned teacher was while I was subbing a led Ashtanga Yoga class because I needed the money. I spent the whole class rolling my eyes over all the seated forward bends (which I blamed for the miserable state of my hamstrings) and telling off Pattabhi Jois in my head for inappropriately touching his female students while adjusting them. Yes, I was also most definitely triggered by this. So when one student asked for a forceful adjustment in order to get into a deeper hamstring stretch, I said no and proceeded to go on a small rant about connective tissue, passive ranges of motion, and consent. My outburst had nothing to do with teaching anyone in the class anything, it was me telling these poor folks, who just wanted to move and breathe a little, that what they were doing was wrong. My feelings of frustration were valid but at the head of a classroom was not an appropriate place to vent them. In retrospect, the nastiest part of the disillusionment stage was that it was impossible to keep my confusing, turbulent inner process out of my teaching. It's damn hard to ground yourself when you feel like the foundation beneath your feet is crumbling.

So, when an opportunity came my way to quit teaching, I took it. With a whole lotta bitterness I rolled up my yoga mat and headed out to the middle of nowhere to be a wildfire lookout. Screw community, I wanted to be alone. I knew others who felt similar about yoga, but I still felt isolated in my critiques. Part of me also worried that those in the yoga community who dismissed my critical social media presence as "negative" and "not believing in myself" were true. At this point, I'd been critical for years and it hadn't brought me any clarity.

I found very little joy in yoga anymore, but I still kind of loved yoga. I knew there was still something great to be had in its practices so I couldn't give it up. It was akin to living in a perpetual state of feeling like I'd just shat my spiritual bed. And so, I promised myself that if after a five month break from it all if I never wanted to teach/practice again, I'd quit for good. I didn't read about yoga, I didn't get into online debates, I didn't post practice pictures or updates, I unfollowed yoga teachers on social media whose posts made me feel like negative-vibed crap. I'd say I "let it go" but the truth is that idealistic sense of antagonism stayed heavy on my shoulder every time I went for a walk, climbed my lookout ladder, or took a less than optimal poo.

Angry, Special People

Disillusioned teaching is a little like authoritarian teaching only instead of the answer being, "I'm right and you're wrong," it's, "That's bullshit and no, I don't know what the right answer is. What's wrong with you people?" Other common phrases or internal dialogue might include:

"I used to love wide angle forward bends...before they broke my ass and the teacher told me that the ripping sound was my hips opening."

"Heart openers? What? Like there's a zipper on your sternum or something?"

"Solve your own problems." *usually muttered under breath

"Can you sub for me tonight?"

I wouldn't say disillusionment feels good, but there is a perverse sort of enjoyment to be had in cynicism and indignation. It's almost punk rock. Our anger fuels our teaching and becomes a way to feel grounded and legit in a world of perceived phonies. God, I loved feeling legit in a world of phonies. I loved finding other legit people to make fun of all the phonies with. I also loved feeling a little more legit than those new friends. Rebellion is a grand thing, but we can only get so far defining ourselves by what we are not. As Billy-Joel

Armstrong of Green Day once said, "Being an angry young man is sexy but no one likes a bitter old bastard." When we marry our sense of identity to forever being the defiant outsider, we can end up painting ourselves into an ideological corner. If we don't give ourselves room to change and progress, we'll end up just as burnt-out as when we started, but with a little extra indignation thrown in. So what I propose is this: disillusionment is a necessary process to move through, not an identity to get stuck in.

Your Story: Run Out of Good Vibes?

How has your view of yoga (practice, community, business, everything) changed since you started practicing?

How do you currently reconcile the seemingly conflicting information on yoga's past, present, and future? Do you bypass certain issues to avoid inner conflict? How might this bypassing affect yourself and others?

What's your experience with disillusionment and burnout? How did your teaching change during this experience? Good, bad, and ugly. If you don't have any, how do you feel about it potentially happening one day? Do you think disillusionment is something to be avoided or embraced?

How has the identity of being disillusioned and/or rebellious affected you as a teacher and as a practitioner? Is this a self-identification or a label that has been put on you? If you experience the latter, how does it affect how you feel about and interact with the broader yoga community?

Has manipulation, elitism, bullying, and poor boundaries played a part in your becoming disillusioned with mainstream yoga? Talk about the experience (get as angry as you need to).

Has discrimination and bias within yoga communities played a part in your becoming disillusioned with mainstream yoga? Talk about the experience (get as angry as you need to).

Has the commodification of yoga and the business side of being a yoga teacher played a part in your becoming disillusioned with mainstream yoga? Talk about the experience (get as angry as you need to).

Anything else you want to say about disillusionment?

Practice Discernment and Refinement

Let Yourself Feel Stuff

Back to me, alone and bitter, in the middle of nowhere. I didn't even practice for the first two or three months. I still thought about yoga a lot, and felt a lot of things about the impact it had had on my life, but there was less pressure to turn any of my process into a performance for a class or social media. Eventually, partially due to my bum knee acting up, I started practicing again. I don't know exactly why or how I decided to pick yoga back up, pilates would have been just as good for my knee, I just legitimately wanted to practice. Instead of a burden, it felt freeing again—something it hadn't been for years. I even started thinking about teaching again and liking the thought of it. But it was different, there was a personal resolve grounding my yoga that, up until that point, I had never possessed as a teacher. I had let myself feel all those shit feelings about the yoga world without making them the basis of my personal practice, and, in doing so, they helped refine what yoga was for me and what it wasn't. I sat with all the shame and discomfort of my past mistakes and began to feel twinges of self-compassion, and eventually even self-forgiveness. I know, I know, I was practicing yoga to rediscover yoga. How cliché (disillusioned yoga Tori would have called all this complete bullshit). But upon closer examination, that process wasn't just yoga, it was grief.

What I think is often overlooked is that disillusionment is part of a grieving process. Finding out that our cure-all for being human is not what it seemed, realizing that we were perhaps put-on by those who sold it to us, seeing Indigenous cultures repeatedly misrepresented, appropriated and dumbed down to sell products (especially if it's your culture!) is hard. Really hard. Infuriating even. Choosing to not play a role in any of it anymore can mean a loss of job security, income, and possibly community. It also means, for many of us, taking full responsibility for the role we have played in perpetuating this harmful mess. Having a whole lotta feelings to work through about all that seems pretty normal to me. If we don't take the time needed to feel and grieve, we risk becoming stuck in bitterness and/or bypassing for the sake of looking like, "one of the good ones."

Grief teaching can be a little like going on a date with someone who's recently divorced and is attempting to "get back out there" way too soon. We're trying our best, but our heart is still hurting and we are not sure what we want. This is okay. We can't all take five months off teaching to grieve and self-reflect alone in the woods— sometimes we have to process in front of others, awkward as it may be. In fact, I'd say this clumsiness can be part of our healing—a transparent, non bypassed step in our growth as yoga practitioners. We are allowed to acknowledge we are both teachers and humans, remember?

We may never forgive some of what's been done to us, those we care about, and to itself in the name of so-called yoga, and we don't have to, but we can forgive ourselves. I forgive myself, past and present, all the time. Personally, forgiveness is a pressure valve for releasing the shame that would have me pointing fingers at every other yoga teacher on the planet as a way of escaping my own conscience. I still disagree with a lot of what goes on in the name of yoga but my goal in speaking out is not to dis-identify with the issues or my role in perpetuating them—it's about knowing what my yoga practice is and what it stands for.

Growing Pains

Every religion (the analogy works regardless of whether or not you view your yoga practice as religious) has its born-again stage when everything is new and shiny and it's going to solve all of my problems and your problems and everybody else's problems—if only everyone would listen to me. This stage cannot last if we continue to deepen our understanding of that to which we have committed ourselves. As our understanding deepens, we will inevitably start to question and change our beliefs and behaviours. We will also start to question the beliefs and behaviours of those around us. This isn't a new process to yoga—many ancient sages, such as Vyasa, wrote about different stages of knowing (Yoga-Bhashya, 3.51). We can't be both innocent and wise, and the cost of wisdom is usually discomfort. And so begins our yoga crisis.

Disillusionment is a step on the path towards developing discernment (*viveka* in Sanskrit). It's how we mature from blind faith to critical thought, which is not the absence of trust but a way to strengthen and deepen it. When our reliance on dogmatic easy answers begins to lessen, we become better able to apply critical thought and deliberation to what we study. This is not us being critical or negative, it's asking the questions that refine our understanding of what it is we do. Cultural appropriation, for example, is not a binary right/wrong condition to get freaked out over, it's an ongoing discussion worth having. Or, even the content of this book—nothing I write here should be taken as gospel. This book is a whole bunch of ideas and practices I hope you will mull over, make up your own mind about, and apply where relevant.

What we initially saw as a crisis can become our new normal. I sometimes call this "living in the grey areas." This is a mindset that promotes every question as valid, looks at new ideas, revisits old ideas, and doesn't get hung-up on what's shiny and new but also doesn't disqualify something simply because it's shiny and new. In case I made all that sound pretentious and grand, make no mistake—the shift from blind adherence to mindful discernment is awkward, full of screw-ups, and can feel like trying to solve a comedically large, impossibly complicated Rubik's cube while at the same time teaching someone else how to solve it.

The hardest part to come to terms with about this shift is that, in order to maintain it, we have to become better equipped at being uncomfortable. Refinement is not about always feeling good. It's also not about continuous rebellion or jumping to the next new trend and/or teaching identity. We tried teaching yoga for the sake of feeling good all the time and it didn't work. If you're anything like me it could make you teach rather badly and, in the long run, feel worse. There's so much more available to us if we're willing to simply give up the easy answers and begin asking better questions.

We can still love yoga and at the same time be sad about discovering the horrible things that have been done in the name of healing others. We can be grateful for what we have gotten from our practice and still acknowledge how that same practice has hurt us. We can find an aspect of the yoga world reprehensible and say so, knowing that sometimes practicing acceptance means accepting that something is unacceptable. Embracing complexity, along with the uncertainty that comes with it, is a sign of a maturing practice.

Your Practice: How Will You Bring Discernment and Refinement into Your Teaching

What do you love about yoga? What do you hate about yoga? Can the two lists above coexist? If they can't, what needs to change in order for that to happen?

What does grief feel like to you? Where and how do you feel it in your body? What you write for this question doesn't need to be a right answer or even make sense. How can you give yourself space to grieve—in your life, practice, and teaching? Can you put what you grieve about yoga into words? If not, maybe a picture, dance, or other form of expression.

In making room for grief, what other emotions are you allowing to surface? How can you skillfully create more space for emotions like anger and sadness in your practice and teaching? (hint: think transparency)

What role can forgiveness play in your yoga practice? Forgiveness of self? Of others? If forgiveness of some people/events is not possible (it's not a requirement for healing), what else do you need in order to move forward with your life and yoga practice?

What are your grey areas, meaning areas where you feel conflicted and confused about yoga? Don't be shy—we all have them. This question isn't about solving these things, just acknowledging they exist and owning them.

If dogma and easy answers are no longer the foundation of your yoga, what is? Start by brainstorming a list of qualities you want to embody in the world as a yogi. Take the top three that are most important to you and explain how you intend to practice and uphold these. What do you want your yoga to stand for? How does it feel to know and articulate this?

How does practicing discernment and critical thought look for you? Remember, it's praxis in practice, not something we get right.

Back to Doubt Again: Imposter Syndrome and Perfectionism

And here we all are back at doubt again. Yay.

This whole book is kind of about doubt, or, rather, how we try to avoid it. I didn't intend that. It just happened while I was writing it and made a whole lot of sense. When you strip away all the ways we bypass and avoid, what's left is usually messy and terrifying. Most of us started doing yoga because we wanted to feel better. Most of us became yoga teachers because we wanted to keep the feeling-better ball rolling. The problem is that yoga is not about feeling better. Yes, it can change our lives, but nowhere in any sutra does it claim to make all of life's troubles go away; there is no sutra anywhere that makes mention of "Good Vibes Only."

When I stopped faking, bullying, and bitching, what I found was a very scared person in overpriced stretchy pants. Seven years of experience and multiple trainings and I felt like I knew nothing. I found myself worried about what and how I was teaching all the time. Was it too hard? Was it too easy? Too spiritual or not spiritual enough? Did that person who came to my class really like it or were they just being nice? I kept studying and learning but gaining more knowledge did nothing to quell my fears. I'd freeze up in class and have a hard time being present with who I was teaching. I dreaded posting yoga videos on social media because I was sure someone would find something wrong with them/me. I really wanted to not care about any of it but the more I tried to just be cool, the more I felt like a fraud. It was exhausting.

The most debilitating part of it all was knowing that none of it was real, but for the life of me I couldn't stop believing it.

During this time, a more experienced teacher and friend, a great friend, used to come to my classes sometimes. Every single time it was like everyone else in the room disappeared, and not in a good way. I'd watch her every move for a sign of discontent or disapproval. When I wasn't overcompensating with planks and charm, I'd be dumbfounded as to what to say, because what wisdom did I have to offer someone who had once been my teacher? I knew deep down that I had something to offer, but it was always just out of reach. Never quite there and never quite as it should be. It was like one of those alignment cues that doesn't quite make sense; picture yourself between two panes of glass and then freak out because you're trapped between two panes of glass. Whatever it was that was missing, if I could just get it, really get it, then I'd finally be a great teacher.

"It" was being perfect. Well, whatever I thought perfect was. No, that's not right. I wanted what I thought everyone else saw as perfect. For most of my twenties I'd affirmed to myself that, "I was enough," but I never stopped to consider just what I was affirming I was enough of. For most of my thirties I did an apparent 360 degree switch to celebrating my imperfection, but that turned out to be the new trend of how to be perfect. What is perfectionism? Well, it's this insidious and ridiculous idea that there is only one best way to be human. Only one. Sounds silly when I put it like that, right? It is, but as an unspoken belief it is a force to be reckoned with. Perfection has power over us because it's so ingrained in our Western society that it's everywhere we turn. It's everywhere you look in Westernized yoga; only one best way to look, act, speak, move, teach, succeed, eat, defecate, and fuck. These long established social ideals have become so normalized that we buy into them without even realizing it. And, it's a lie. An unattainable, unjustifiable lie that, if believed, will keep us running ourselves down forever.

Perfectionism, what a fucking asshole.

But Am I Really a Good Teacher?

Imposter syndrome is the feeling that we are somehow ill-equipped or under-qualified for the work we do. It's similar to self-doubt, but it's more professionally specific; we don't think we are good at what we do, or, at least not as good as someone else (insert teacher you love/hate on Instagram). It commonly shows up as perfectionism because we think being prefect is the only way to not fail at what we are doing.

Please keep in mind that I'm talking about all this as it relates to teaching. I'm not a therapist specializing in anxiety disorder, trauma, systems of oppression, or anything else that can contribute to imposter syndrome in the broader sense. Though, I know enough to say that these factors absolutely contribute. So, while what I talk about and suggest here can help us learn to be more comfortable as a teacher, it is not the answer to everything.

The hardest part of imposter syndrome is that we lose our gauge for what's real and what isn't. Any discernment skills we've cultivated fly out the window when it comes to our own capabilities; "I did that well, but was it good enough?" I mention the amount of trainings I've completed throughout the book not to brag but to prove a point—more trainings are not only not always indicative of wisdom, and they often aren't the answer to imposter syndrome. More knowledge, both theoretical and experiential, is great, but it's not going to stop our insecurity sweats when we don't have the ability to measure our own professional worth.

We can intellectually know that our perfectionist-driven insecurities are ridiculous and still believe that we are missing the mark more than everyone else. In this situation, we can easily fall into behaviours that are not about good teaching, but an attempt to hide our fear and insecurity. We can know better and still fall into using ill-advised safety blankets like sexuality and manipulation that we can wrap ourselves in to feel safe and secure. For me, looking back there was an idea that if I could trick people into thinking I was perfect, then maybe someday I'd actually get there. Unfortunately, my tricks and performances had the pesky side effect of making my imposter syndrome even worse. I know "fake it until you make it" works for some people but all it ever did for me was make me better at faking.

A long-term consequence of using any of the unadvisable teaching strategies we've explored here is that we will never really be seen for who we are by those we teach. The consequences of never being seen for who we are is that we will always feel like an imposter, because, frankly, we are an imposter. It's a cycle we are taught and, in many cases sold, and it is a terrifying way to teach, and live. If we teach in a way that is not in line with who we really are as person— good, bad and ugly—we'll feel like a fake. Not because what we're teaching is bad, but because we can't trust ourselves to recognize it.

Your Story: Terrified Much?

What's your experience of imposter syndrome and self-doubt? What does it feel like in your body? How do you usually respond? What coping mechanisms do you use?

What are the pros and cons of perfectionism, in your own life and in yoga?

In what areas of yoga/yoga teaching do you doubt yourself? Why? Which doubts do you think are founded and which are not? Is there any truth in what you think makes you an imposter, or not? Get specific. It helps to know what we actually think about ourselves as teachers and what it's based on.

How can external factors like yoga culture, and our culture at large, contribute to internalized imposter syndrome? Think about advertisements, social media, etc. Give special attention to cultural biases like sexism, ableism, homophobia, and racism.

How do you respond to imposter syndrome and self-doubt in others? Is it similar to how you respond to yourself, of different? Why?

How does perfectionism and/or the belief in perfectionism influence how you teach and how you present yourself as a teacher? If the notion of perfectionism didn't exist, how would your teaching be different?

If you don't use perfectionism to guide your teaching abilities, what else could you use? What else is available to you? Can this be extended to others? Does is change how you view yourself and others?

Any other thoughts, experiences, and/or insights on imposter syndrome and perfectionism?

Practice Self-Trust and Community

Self-Trust Though Action

Self-trust is not an energetic light switch we can turn on. We can have lightbulb moments of clarity about ourselves, but those insights need to be backed up by action if we ever hope to change our patterns. Good intentions are a start, but alone they aren't enough. It's through responsible, accountable actions that we can start to build self-trust. This is the place in the book, you could say, where the rubber really meets the road.

The actions we can start with are the ones we've talked about so far in this book: boundaries, transparency, inclusion, empathy, discernment, and everything else we've gone into. The praxis of applying this new knowledge is how we start to experiment with being seen for who we are and what we know. If you have intense imposter syndrome that likely sounds terrifying, but please bear with me.

Starting to focus on the skills of teaching, instead of teaching being a means to perfecting ourselves, helps us get out of our own heads, namely because it requires us to focus on interacting with people in the room instead of ourselves. It's no longer about us alone at the front of the room, trying to be the teacher we think we should be; teaching yoga becomes about sharing what we know with a group of people with boundaries and aptitude. It sounds a lot simpler than being *insert preferred deity again*, doesn't it? Take out the burden of an identity crutch, and teaching yoga gets a lot simpler.

To break it down:

1. Becoming more transparent about who we are, in addition to making us a more effective teacher, helps us determine the boundaries we need as a teacher.

2. Determining and unapologetically setting emotional/interpersonal/professional boundaries helps us to feel safe as a teacher because we are aware and honest about what we need, what we know, and what is out of bounds.

3. Feeling safe enables us to show up, practice discernment, and take more responsibility for ourselves because we are less freaked-out (I like to think of professional scope as a big soft safety bubble that grows with me over time).

4. Taking responsibility for ourselves motivates and empowers us to notice our blind spots and adverse teaching tactics and, hopefully, do something about them as required.

5. Over time, seeing ourselves actively be responsible and capable proves to us that we are accountable. Accountability fosters professional trust in ourselves, our skills, and our capacity to grow and learn even more.

6. That builds confidence. At long last, a real confidence, not based on tricks or overcompensation, but a solid trust based on showing up for ourselves and seeing what we are capable of with no need to delude ourselves or anyone else.

Yes, it's a process that takes time. There's nothing wrong with that. Please remember that accountability isn't self-shaming, its loving ourselves enough to take a long hard look at our actions.

And are any of these practices going to be perfect? Of course not. Are they perfect for everyone? OF COURSE NOT. Are we going to mess up any of them as badly as we think? Probably not. Are we still going to have the odd day with panic sweats? Most likely. It doesn't mean we're failing at any of it, just that we are learning something new. Every skill and attitude we've covered overlaps with one another in such a way that real growth in any one area requires a slow and steady growth in all. This seems like an opportune time to remind you that I had to relearn all of this ten years after I had a degree in it. Experiential learning, i.e. the good stuff, is always a bit on the messy side.

Healthy Community

We can only grow so far doing it alone. Trust me, I've tried.

Sussing out blind-spots and being accountable all on our own usually amounts to chasing our own perfectionist tail. For me, I have opted for a mix of personal and professional support. I have a therapist, I have teachers, I have yoga teacher peers (in person and online), I have peers that have no interest in yoga, and I am lucky to have my family. The hands-down best way to begin being okay with being ourselves when we teach, is by being okay with being ourselves in our lives. Acceptance is personal, but it's also very much a communal practice. In all honesty, it's all communal practice. Which brings us to the value of community. It's not a social work best practice but it's invaluable none the less.

You know that teacher friend who made me want to vomit whenever she came to my class? Well, at her gentle nudging, we started talking about my imposter syndrome fears which, much to my surprise, she could relate to. Turns out there's always another senior teacher/person/expert to freak out about, no matter how long you've been teaching. There's also always going to be someone who doesn't like the way you teach. The perfect yoga teacher doesn't exist, because everyone wants and needs something different from yoga. There really is no such thing as perfection in yoga, there's only preference.

My friend and I also started talking about manipulation, disillusionment, dogma, business ethics and everything else on our minds. Our aim wasn't (and still isn't) to fix ourselves, each other, or yoga, but to simply talk about everything that has the potential to isolate us from each other and our community. Remember in the saviourism section when I talked about the value of simply being present with people? Well, the value of that is also true in personal relationships. Healthy relationships and communities never grow out of us trying to fix/heal one another. Attempting to fix others can temporarily make us feel like a valuable community member but in the long run it alienates us from others, and ourselves. It's nearly impossible to practice presence and acceptance while acting on the compulsion to correct everything we perceive as wrong—this is perfectionism sneaking back in under the guise of healing. Holding space for our friends, just as they are, and allowing them to hold space for us, just as we are, is community at its best in my opinion. Being seen and being heard by our community is a healing balm for imposter syndrome's self-inflicted wounds.

An example of a more structured form of community support in my life is a gathering another friend of mine hosts. There's usually food and socializing before we sit in a circle and voluntarily share whatever we need to share—triumphs and challenges. The key is that no one interrupts you, offers you advice, or says anything apart from, "I see you and thank you for sharing." We don't talk about anything anyone else shares outside of the circle. All we do is hold space for one another to speak; that is more than enough. It's also free, apart from donations to cover costs, not part of anyone's business or marketing plan, and is not exclusive to anyone. Subjective opinion alert: community is best when it's not also a business venture.

Now, all this talk about acceptance doesn't mean we don't also owe it to our community to hold each other accountable when need be. Back to my friend and I, our willingness to simply be present with one another has, over the years, allowed us to cultivate a relationship where hard conversations, and even call-outs, can be honest and safe. It's not me getting chastised for falling short, it's a conversation with someone who accepts and loves me enough to talk about a harmful blind spot I couldn't see myself. And I do the same for her because, as we all now know, social influence goes both ways in healthy relationships. It's not about fixing anyone; it's about learning and relearning from each other for our mutual benefit and shared liberation. Remember, expertise, like acceptance, is a communal practice.

Now, it's easy to read all of this, agree, and then go right back to feeling like we're all alone and still suck. *That is why having friends and community to remind us is so bloody essential.* I remind my friends when they forget, and they do the same for me. No shame. No guilt. No perfection. Self-love is a beautiful ideal but I've never met anyone who didn't occasionally need a reminder that they're worthy and loved just as they are. Without those reminders, it's a slippery slope from practicing accountability into self-flagellation. There's no doubt in my mind that, without the acceptance and love shown to me by my community, in person and online, I would have ever had the courage to tell the stories I have in this book. I don't feel ashamed of any of it, by the way. Remorse, sure, but I know my worth isn't measured by past mistakes. Solid community taught me that.

Your Practice: How Will You Bring Self-Trust Community Into Your Practice and Teaching

Review everything you listed under "Stuff I Know A Lot About" in the professional boundaries section. Look at this list of skills and check-in with how you feel. No right or wrong, it's just good to know how you relate to your own skills. List at least one instance for each where you used this skill/knowledge as a teacher to benefit someone and feel proud of yourself for how you did it. Go into detail. Own it.

Looking at the areas where maybe your doubts are founded, have you ever done anything to advance your knowledge in this area? Why or why not? What are some reasonable steps you could take to learn more about these areas you're interested in?

Do you talk about your doubts and imposter syndrome with anyone? Is this something you think would help you? If so, how can you make it more of a professional priority?

How can accountability be a part of your practice and teaching? How can you build it into what you do as a way of creating confidence and self-trust? What are the tangible steps and what are the broad intentions?

Name three people you know who you feel like you can be yourself around or could be yourself around and who you feel supported by. They can be yoga friends or not. Are these people a priority in your life? Why or why not? If not, what can you do reach out and connect more with them?

How would you like to be supported as a yoga teacher? How can you help create environments for this support? How can you support other yoga teachers?

How can you help to grow communal expertise and acceptance in your yoga community? How can this help promote accountability? How can you safeguard yourself from falling into fixing and perfectionism? If/when you do fall into these old patterns, how can you get yourself out? (hint: you don't have to do it alone)

How To Teach Yoga: That Whole "True Self" Thing

To put it simply, this is how you teach yoga:

Your knowledge of yoga + you + self awareness = you teaching yoga.

Your knowledge of yoga is going to change and grow and contradict itself for as long as you are teaching. We will all inevitably look back in a few years and think, "I was teaching *that?* What was I thinking?" So there's no sense in worrying ourselves sick over it. Only be worried if you look back in a few years and your style of teaching and knowledge haven't changed at all. We can't know everything, but we can share what we have to offer. That's all we can ask of ourselves or anyone else.

You, in all your uniquely you wonderfulness, are who you are. Parts of you are amazing and parts of you are cruddy. Things about you may change and other things may stay blessedly, or annoyingly, the same. This is part of being a human being, and nowhere in any wisdom tradition does it say that the way to becoming a good teacher is to deny this. Work through parts of it, sure, but denial doesn't get us anywhere. So, you might as well just be who you are—even when you're not entirely sure who that is. The characteristics of your life will also shift and change. Your opinions, lifestyle, life outlooks, personal practice, confidence, health, family situation, finances, and everything else about you will most likely not stay the same as you continue to teach. All of the above make up who you are as a unique individual. None of the above make you a bad teacher. What can trip us up is not being aware of how our personal lives, experiences, and needs can impact our teaching. This is the value of self-awareness as a teacher.

Self-awareness, like everything in yoga, is a practice that will never be perfect. While ideally we'd all subscribe to understand the ancient texts and practices to the extent that we would have ultimate self awareness, this is not the reality for any of us. I think it's realistic to say that we'll all likely have blind spots as long as we're alive. This is why I'm such an advocate for the practices and attitude shifts outlined in this book; they are all tools to diminish the likelihood that our blind spots will do us or anyone else harm. Think of them as ahimsa (non-harming) safeguards for everyone involved. Safeguards that allow everyone to grow, change, learn, and flourish in their own unique way.

Your Best Practices:

One more time, if you please. For each of the following, jot down a few points about what this practice means to you and how you envision integrating it into in your teaching (I suggest starting simple and doable). Yes, they're in a new order:

Professional Boundaries and Scope:

Interpersonal/relationship Boundaries:

Emotional Boundaries:

Transparency:

Humility:

Inclusion:

Appreciation vs. Appropriation:

Empathy:

Autonomy:

Discernment:

Self-trust:

Community:

Anything else that's important for you personally:

Look over the above lists and, to each one, add how you will show yourself compassion while attempting to apply this new practice (that goes double if you really want to skip this step).

Congratulations! Everything you just wrote is YOUR best practices model for teaching yoga.

This is the model of how you would like to show up as a teacher. In practice it will not always turn out the way you'd like but you know what you're aiming for. Remember that whole, "teaching yoga is hard" bit? Well, unlearning how we teach yoga so we can do better is also hard. It'll get awkward at times and that's okay. I still catch myself saying old-school teacher phrases I dislike such as, "Play" in class, despite all my convictions not too. Habits die hard. We'll also get it wrong with the best of intentions, and that's okay too. When I first decided to teach with less authority, I went so far in the opposite direction that I refused to tell anyone anything definitive for fear it would somehow damage them. We'll think we have it down and then find out we had no idea what we were doing. I look at it all this way, all those missteps and imperfect actions are a sure sign I'm not bypassing the real work, and not bypassing is something to feel delightfully confident about.

The real gift of cultivating professional self-trust as a yoga teacher is the ability to separate our emotional fluctuations from our abilities. I can have a bad day and yoga doesn't need to fix it. I can feel bad about myself and still be a freakin 'amazing yoga teacher. Someone can dislike both me and my class, but I still know I have good things to offer. My teaching is no longer about me feeling good about myself, because I have other tools with which to gauge my abilities. I will likely have self-doubt until the day I die, but cultivating professional self-trust is how I stopped believing I had to be perfect. And that's my hope for you; not that you get any of this right but that you are able to be yourself without shame, teach what you want with clarity, and value whoever is in front of you.

Happy teaching.

Om Shanti.

Afterword

Oh wow, not only did you read to the end of the book, but you're also reading the additional snippet at the end? You, my friend, are a champ. I hope you enjoyed reading it. Honestly, I didn't always enjoy writing it, but labours of love are like that. I have cherished this book from its humble beginnings as a too-long Instagram rant all the way to approving copy-edits and finding I STILL had no understanding of semicolons. It's been an uncomfortable labour of love from start to finish.

If you got this copy of the book for free or on loan from someone, I want you to know that you and I are still cool. Personally, I think the monetary ratio of what most teachers make per class compared to the average price of a yoga related training is a bit ridiculous. So, if you need to save money, I understand, and I'm still impressed you read all the way to the snippet at the end.

If you're a yoga teacher or a yoga teacher trainer and are interested in incorporating some of my ideas into your courses, I'm all for it. I just ask that you please do so with respect for the two years it took to write this book and the decade and a half it took to live the lessons within it.

If you use my work or ideas, please reference me as the source. If you want to use my content as part of a training you facilitate, please reach out to me and we'll work out an arrangement that benefits us both. Yes, this is an ask for professional boundaries and staying within your lane in regard to my work. Your stories and your reflections are your own, share with as many or as few people as your boundaries allow.

Thanks, I appreciate it.

Tori

People To Follow and Learn From

This is a very small look at who's out there when it comes to people and perspectives that can help make us better yoga teachers. Please think of this list as an introduction to going down the rabbit hole of alternatives to the dominant yoga norm—a place to start rather than stop. Everyone on this list is described using their own words as much as possible.

Accessible Yoga - a nonprofit organization dedicated to removing barriers that prevent marginalized people from benefiting from yoga. Annual conference, online academy, and weekly podcast, Accessible Yoga podcast. accessibleyoga.org

Allé K (they/he) - yoga teacher offering a variety of online classes centring queer, trans, and non-binary people. nonbinaryogi.com

Amber Karnes (she/her) - yoga teacher/trainer focused on body positive yoga and inclusivity. Offers online classes, cohost of the Accessible Yoga podcast, and leads a body positive and accessible teachers trainings. bodypositiveyoga.com

Asha Frost (she/her) - Indigenous teacher and author offering classes in traditional wisdom and appreciating instead of appropriating Indigenous cultures. ashafrost.com

Black Yoga Magazine - a publication dedicated to highlighting the yoga community of colour. blackyogamagazine.com

Cheyenne Leskanic (she/her) - yoga teacher, writer, and founder of
the Three Medicines Longhouse; a community based in circular
wellness through multifaceted Indigenous wellness paradigms.
threemedicineslonghouse.com

Constanza Eliana Chinea (she/her) - specializes in educating yoga
teachers and wellness entrepreneurs on how to decolonize their
practices, create equity for teachers of colour, and build inclusive
spaces. embodyinclusivity.com

Daniel Sannito (they/them) - yoga teacher and self-described "gender
explorer", offering online yoga and meditation classes.
danielsannito.com

Decolonizing Fitness - Ilya (he/they) is a fitness educator whose
work centres racial, gender, and healing justice. Offerings include an
ebook on creating LGBTQIA+ affirming spaces.
decolonizingfitness.com

Decolonizing Practices - online courses designed to stimulate social
change and transform colonial narratives. Founder Ta7talíya Michelle
Nahanee's (she/her) work is grounded in Squamish teachings.
decolonizingpractices.org

Diane Bondy (she/her) - yoga teacher and trainer offering inclusive
online classes and trainings. She is also the leader of the Yoga for All
Movement. www.dianebondyyoga.com

Fringe(ish): Fat Positive Yoga - Shannon (she/they) offers online
yoga and meditation classes that are trauma-sensitive, accessible, fat
positive, and LGBTQSIA+ affirming. fringeish.com

Jesal Parikh (she/her) - Movement educator and yoga teacher
mentor. Co-creator and co-host of the Yoga Is Dead Podcast.
Founder of Yoga Teachers Of Colour. yogawallanyc.com

Jessamyn Stanley (she/they) - inclusive yoga teacher and body positivity advocate. Author of *Every Body Yoga: Let Go Of Fear, Get On The Mat, Love Your Body*, host of Dear Jessamyn Podcast, and primary teacher at The Underbelly online studio. jessamynstanley.com

Jivana Heyman (he/him) - founder of Accessible Yoga and author of *Accessible Yoga: Poses And Practices For Every Body*. Co-host of the Accessible Yoga podcast. accessibleyoga.org

Karen James (she/her) - Black yoga teacher offering online yoga classes and lots of accessible yoga tutorials on her Instagram account. @karenjamesyoga

Karin Carlson (she/her) - yoga teacher/trainer offering an online anti-200-hour training and mentorship program strongly focused on social justice and inclusion. returnyoga.org

Kallie Schut (she/her) - yoga teacher offering online classes and a 10 hour online course; "Decolonizing and Honoring Yoga: Race Equity, Cultural Appropriation, and Integrity." rebelyogatribe.co.uk

Layla F. Saad (she/her) - anti-racist educator, author of *Me And White Supremacy* and host of The Good Ancestor Podcast. laylafsaad.com

Leesa Renee Hall (she/her) - anti-bias and anti-racist facilitator specializing in helping highly sensitive people through reflective writing and self inquiry. Host of the Inner Field Trip podcast. leesareneehall.com

Marc Settembrino (he/they) - educator, researcher, and yoga facilitator offering classes through his online studio, "The Fat Kid Yoga Club." marcsettembrino.com

Manoj Dias (he/him) - a mindfulness and meditation teacher born and raised in the Theravada Buddhist Tradition. Livestream meditation classes available. mnojdias.com.au

Off The Mat - online trainings designed to bridge the gap between yoga and conscious activism. Website has a great list of recommended anti-racism reading material. offthemat.com

Puja Singh Titchkosky (they/them) - yoga/meditation teacher and musician offering a body of work that is informed by and shared through a lens of decolonization and dismantling oppressive systems of power. princepuja.net

Michelle C. Johnson - yoga teacher, activist, and author of "Skill In Action: Radicalizing Your Yoga To Create A Just World." Offers the course "Dismantling Racism" and other online trainings. michellecjohnson.com

Pam Palmater (she/her) – holds a Doctorate in Law. Online videos, blogs, and podcast centres Indigenous education, sovereignty, and nation building. pampalmater.com

The State of Union - a six-part series created by BIPOC (Black, Indigenous, and People of Colour) in the yoga industry, as an act of conscious protest via dialogue. stateofunionyoga.com

Susanna Barkataki (she/her) - yoga teacher/trainer focused on honouring yoga's roots and educating yogi's about cultural appropriation. Offers online yoga trainings, including a masterclass on using the word "Namaste." embraceyogasroots.com

Tristan Katz (they/them) - digital strategist and equity-inclusion facilitator for yoga teachers and healers. Offering include a Social Media and Marketing Workbook. katz-creative.com

Tegal Patel (she/her) - yoga teacher and trainer offering online yoga and meditation classes as well as a BIPOC coaching and mediation circle. Co-creator and co-host of the Yoga Is Dead Podcast. tegalyoga.com

Yoga Teachers of Color- a grassroots movement celebrating diversity in yoga and advocating for representation. yogateachersofcolor.com

Resources

Pandit Arya (1986) *Yoga Sutras Of Patanjali With Exposition By Vyasa,* Himalayan Institute

Susanna Barkataki (2020) *Embrace Yoga's Roots: Courageous Ways to Deepen Your Yoga Practice,* Ignite Yoga and Wellness Institute

A. Cohn, A. Canter - National Association of School Psychologists (2003) *Bullying: Facts for_schools_and parents,* naspcenter.org

Henry Cloud (2002) *Boundaries: When to Say Yes, How to Say No, to Take Control of Your Life,* Zondervan

Frank Cooper (2012) *Professional Boundaries in Social Work and Social Care: A Practical Guide to Understanding, Maintaining and Managing Your Professional Boundaries,* Jessica Kingsley Publishers

Shakil Choudhury (2015) *Deep Diversity: Overcoming Us vs. Them,* Between The Lines

Laura van Dernoot Lipsky (2009) *Trauma Stewardship: An Everyday Guide to Caring for Self While Caring for Others,* Berrett-Koehler Publishers

Paulo Freire (1968) *Pedagogy of the Oppressed,* Bloomsbury Publishing Inc

JD Haltigan, T Vaillancourt - Developmental Psychology (2014) *Joint trajectories of bullying and peer victimization across elementary and middle school and associations with symptoms of psychopathology,* psycnet.apa.org

Kevin K. Kumashiro (2014) *Six Lenses for Anti-Oppressive Education: Partial Stories, Improbable Conversations,* Peter Lang Inc., International Academic Publishers

Kenneth Strike, Jonas Soltis (2009) *The Ethics of Teaching, 5th Edition,* Teachers College Press

About the Author

After two and half decades of spiritual searching, Tori's outlook on life can be summed up simply as, "Just be kind and maybe try therapy." While still a student of Advaita Vedanta, Tori mostly keeps her practice to herself these days.

Tori has a degree in Social Work through the University of Calgary. Though no longer practicing social work in a formal setting, she remains committed to social justice and building healthy communities.

Printed in Great Britain
by Amazon